OSTEOARTHRITIS

PREVENTING AND HEALING WITHOUT DRUGS

OSTEOARTHRITIS

PREVENTING AND HEALING WITHOUT DRUGS

PETER BALES, MD, MHSA

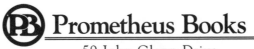 **Prometheus Books**

59 John Glenn Drive
Amherst, New York 14228-2119

Published 2008 by Prometheus Books

Inquiries should be addressed to
Prometheus Books
59 John Glenn Drive
Amherst, New York 14228–2119
VOICE: 716–691–0133, ext. 210
FAX: 716–691–0137
WWW.PROMETHEUSBOOKS.COM

12 11 10 09 08   5 4 3 2 1

Library of Congress Cataloging-in-Publication Data

Bales, Peter, 1962–
    Osteoarthritis : preventing and healing without drugs / by Peter Bales.
        p. cm.
    Includes bibliographical references and index.
    ISBN 978–1–59102–615–0 (pbk. : alk. paper)
    1. Osteoarthritis—Alternative treatment. I. Title.
    [DNLM: 1. Osteoarthritis—etiology. 2. Osteoarthritis—prevention & control.
3. Osteoarthritis—diet therapy. WE 348 B184o 2008].

RC931.O67B35 2008
616.7'223—dc22

                                                              2008007773

Printed in the United States on acid-free paper

Contents

Preface

My motivation for writing this book is based on the fact that a large number of scientific discoveries are occurring daily, but they are slow to be implemented in the daily practice of medicine. A lot of this information is dispersed among different specialties and medical disciplines, but it has not been integrated by organized medicine to the point where it can benefit actual patients. Furthermore, physicians who are at the front lines in treating people with osteoarthritis do not have knowledge of many of the latest discoveries. As a result, many people will not be made aware of this information by consulting their physicians. Another factor complicating the matter is that medicine, as it is currently practiced, is focused on drug treatments and invasive and surgical procedures. The research I will outline in this book focuses on a more holistic approach to treating and preventing osteoarthritis. There is a lack of incorporation of new medical knowledge and treatments into the everyday treatment of patients with osteoarthritis. This information gap in the treatment of osteoarthritis leads arthritis sufferers to seek alternative and complementary medicine more than any other group of patients with degenerative disease.

The research presented in this book has been performed at the most prestigious universities and medical institutions around the world, but these findings have not, for the most part, been incorporated by traditional medical practitioners in the treatment of their patients. It is this knowledge gap that my book aims to fill. After all, knowledge is power!

I was trained at traditional medical universities and am a practicing, board-certified orthopedic surgeon. The inspiration to write this book came from the growing epidemic of osteoarthritis plaguing younger people, which I encounter on a daily basis in my practice. In the past, osteoarthritis was typically associated with the elderly. However, more recently it is plaguing people starting in their thirties. Why? The answer lies in large part to our highly inflammatory diet, consisting in part of our overwhelming consumption of sugar and unhealthy fats. This type of diet has detrimental effects on our health. This will be further discussed in chapters 8, 10, and 11. This book explains how we can "turn on and off" genes in our joints to avoid this crippling disease.

Traditional medicine has a limited number of treatments for osteoarthritis. These include anti-inflammatory medications (which can cause serious side effects), addicting painkillers, and drastic total joint replacement surgery. This book's mission is to provide knowledge and insight on new "alternative" means to treat osteoarthritis without medications or surgery. My extensive research has shown that many recent scientific studies support my theory. These new genetic and nutritional studies are destined to revolutionize the treatment of osteoarthritis. *The new genetic research shows that the same poor nutrition that causes inflammation, obesity, diabetes, and heart disease is also fueling the development of joint deterioration.*

Osteoarthritis affects more than 20 million Americans and is the most common degenerative disorder in the United States. The recent explosion of conditions such as obesity, metabolic syndrome, and diabetes is fueling the increase in joint deterioration and osteoarthritis. The culprit: elevated blood sugar levels, caused by insulin resistance and unhealthy fat consumption, which increase the inflammatory state of our bodies and "turn on" genes that promote the breakdown of cartilage in our joints. Metabolic syndrome, which is associated with obesity, high cholesterol levels, and high blood sugar levels, is estimated to affect 47 million Americans. Unless the current trends are reversed, according to some estimates, one out of four children born in the year 2000 is destined to develop diabetes. These metabolic trends are causing an increase in osteoarthritis and other degenerative diseases in the United States—and, if left unchecked, will bankrupt our ailing healthcare system.

This book is divided into six parts. In part 1, I discuss the impact of osteoarthritis on society and how osteoarthritis leads to cartilage destruction in joints. I then discuss the interrelated metabolic conditions that predispose us to the development of osteoarthritis. These include insulin resistance (pre-diabetes), oxidative stress (decaying process), inflammation, metabolic syndrome, and obesity.

Part 2 outlines the latest research in nutrition and arthritis, which shows how these predisposing metabolic imbalances lead to the development of osteoarthritis. In chapter 9, I discuss the beneficial effects of the "good" fats and omega 3s on our joints. In chapter 10, I discuss how hormonal imbalances caused by obesity and unhealthy diets increases inflammation in joint cartilage. In chapter 11, I discuss how increased sugar in our diets leads to the increased "rusting" of our joints. In chapter 12, I discuss specific side effects of current osteoarthritis drugs and also the potential pitfalls of new drugs that are in the pipeline.

In part 3, I discuss the joint nutrients that have been shown by the latest research to be the most beneficial in combating osteoarthritis. In chapter 13, I discuss how new genetic research is unraveling many chemical substances involved in the development of osteoarthritis. In chapter 14, I discuss a number of beneficial nutrients and vitamins that emerging research has shown to be beneficial to people with osteoarthritis. In chapter 15, I discuss in more detail a comprehensive nutritional arsenal that can be used to combat osteoarthritis. I also discuss two well-known nutraceuticals, **glucosamine** and **chondroitin**, and I detail a number of international scientific studies that support their use in pain control and halting the progression of osteoarthritis.

Part 4 outlines my dietary recommendations for osteoarthritis based on the most current genetic and nutritional research. These include maintaining an optimal weight of BMI less than 25, maintaining low blood sugar levels, increasing the amount of omega-3 fats consumed in the diet, and using nutritional supplements.

In part 5, I discuss how the new basic science research findings support the emergence of a new paradigm in treating degenerative diseases such as osteoarthritis. I discuss the reasons why the old paradigm of using drugs such as painkillers, anti-inflammatories, and steroids is not working to prevent and treat osteoarthritis.

Finally, in part 6, I look to the future, discussing the emerging research fields of nutritional genetics, proteomics (the study of the interaction of proteins with nutrients), and metabolomics (the study of how nutrients improve our metabolism), which will improve our treatments and lead to a cure of osteoarthritis.

We are a knowledge-based society. Scientific knowledge doubles every three to five years! No one person or scientific discipline is the repository of the "holy grail" of knowledge in diseases. People must access information from a variety of sources and be able to synthesize this information to make the best decisions for their health and that of their families. It is in this spirit that I write this book, and I hope it provides a fresh approach to attacking this crippling disease.

Introduction

Osteoarthritis: What It Is and Its Impact on Society

Osteoarthritis affects more than 20 million Americans and it is the most common degenerative disease in the United States.[1] The number of joint replacements performed each year for arthritis in this country is skyrocketing: by the year 2030 it is expected that 3.5 million knee replacements will be performed each year, an increase of 673 percent from current levels.[2] My aim in this book is to address the explosion of osteoarthritis. I will describe the new advances in basic scientific research that point to innovative new solutions to the osteoarthritis crisis. I will then provide concrete recommendations to help people fight this disease.

A number of conditions are fueling the osteoarthritis epidemic. One of these conditions is **obesity**, which affects all age groups and has been scientifically proven to accelerate the development of osteoarthritis. Another is a group of physical risk factors known collectively as **metabolic syndrome**, which is characterized by a large amount of fat around the waist, hypertension, high blood sugar levels, and high cholesterol and triglyceride levels. This dangerous collection of symptoms is a factor in the development of a number of degenerative diseases, including osteoarthritis. It is estimated that 25 percent of all American adults—a whopping 47 million people—have metabolic syndrome.[3] According to some estimates that figure rises to 40 percent in those sixty to sixty-nine years of age.[4] The reason for this epidemic can be traced to a diet consisting of synthetic toxic fats, laboratory-made high-concentration "fructose and corn syrup" found in many foods, and the use of addictive "taste-enhancing" chemicals in packaged foods. The overall message here is that one out of every four people meet the criteria for obesity, elevated blood sugar levels, and increased **inflammation**, all of which negatively affect their health. In the following chapters I will discuss the newest research into the best methods to combat metabolic syndrome and its destructive effects on the body.

When one eats a meal, the body breaks down the food into more basic units, such as protein amino acids, sugars, and fatty acids. These basic units are then converted into energy within the **cells**. This process of converting food into energy is referred to as **metabolism**. Similar to a car burning gas in order to run its engine, the burning of foods in the body creates toxic byproducts. In the case of the car exhaust, CO_2 and ozone are created; in the case of cells, toxic substances are produced that must be eliminated by the body. When these toxins are few, the body is efficient in eliminating them, but when toxins accumulate they cause damage in the cells, which is referred to as **oxidative stress**. Toxins accumulate in the body because the detoxification enzymes (found in the liver and other organs) become overwhelmed and start to malfunction when confronted with many toxic substances in our food (such as bad trans fats) and in our environment (such as pesticides, mercury, and other harmful chemicals). The **detoxification enzyme systems** I will be discussing later are a major means the body has of processing the myriad of chemical substances we come into contact with every day. This oxidative stress in cartilage cells builds up and leads to osteoarthritis. What, then, increases the oxidative stress in our bodies? Known culprits include a bad diet filled with unhealthy fats and sugars, exposure to polluted air and water, exposure to industrial chemicals and food additives, overeating, lack of exercise, and a sedentary lifestyle.

Another important risk factor is increased **body inflammation** caused by eating the wrong types of foods containing high levels of sugars and unhealthy trans fats and **saturated fats**. Diet is a major cause of excessive inflammation in the body, and this inflammation is linked to life-threatening conditions such as heart disease, Alzheimer's disease, and osteoarthritis. Inflammation and oxidative stress work hand in hand to damage our joints, so we must actively prevent their occurrence by educating ourselves on proper nutrition and by avoiding toxic foods.

These conditions lead to an unhealthy environment in the body that damages the cartilage in the joints and leads to the development of osteoarthritis. Osteoarthritis is a condition in which the substance that cushions our joints—the **cartilage**—starts to deteriorate and eventually disappears, leaving a painful condition of joint swelling and stiffness. When this progresses to an advanced stage the only treatment is to replace the diseased joint with metal and plastic components referred to as **total joint replacement**. My aim in this book is to discuss ways to prevent and even reverse the destruction of the joints that results from this debilitating disease.

New research into the effects of nutrition on our overall health has revealed that good nutrition is very important in reducing inflammation in the body and limiting the formation of destructive chemical substances that can breakdown cartilage and cause osteoarthritis. I will show that an unhealthy diet has a direct effect on joint cartilage, causing its breakdown. This is carried out by chemicals, either directly in the food or those that are produced in the body as a result of the specific foods eaten, which are able to communicate either harmful or beneficial signals to the genes inside cartilage cells. **Cartilage cells** are the basic units that make up the cushioning substance found in our joints. **Genes** are the basic information storage units in our cells that, much like a master plan, code for all the chemicals and chemical reactions that are needed to carry out life's everyday functions. They do this by each coding and producing a specific protein that has a distinct function to perform in the cell. Unhealthy foods stimulate specific genes inside cartilage cells to overproduce harmful chemicals that actually break down cartilage. Think about it: cartilage cells *themselves* cause the osteoarthritic destruction of the joints when they are stimulated by unhealthy, toxic diets.

People are constantly bombarded by the lure of unhealthy foods. One big culprit is "empty calorie" carbohydrates. This refers to carbohydrates, such as white flour, that have been chemically stripped of their natural vitamins, minerals, and fiber (which are present in whole grains) and simply provide carbohydrate calories that are quickly converted to sugar when they enter the bloodstream. The food industry advertises extensively to sell good-tasting—and unhealthy and often addictive—foods. Fast-food restaurants that sell high-fat and high-sugar meals are a large part of the problem, but schools don't lag far behind in peddling bad food. School lunches are often made up of sugary soft drinks, unhealthy meats, and refined starches with empty calories. According to the American Diabetes Association, poor nutrition is so rampant that one out of every four children born in the year 2000 is at risk of becoming diabetic, unless drastic changes are made.

Osteoarthritis is very nearly an epidemic in the United States today. There is a large body of scientific research that points to high sugar consumption, unhealthy fat consumption, obesity, and high inflammation in the body as the major culprits. In this book I will discuss how optimizing nutrition and lowering risk factors can help to maintain joint health. I will outline the latest **double-blind scientific research** that shows how nutritional intervention can treat and reverse this disease.

The major advances in the treatment of degenerative joint disease in the last twenty years have been primarily in the surgical treatment of diseased joints. Medicine has not been able to offer patients with osteoarthritis many options other than steroids, nonsteroidal drugs, and painkillers. These drugs have serious side effects and do not address the underlying causes of the disease—they merely treat the symptoms. The drugs currently used to treat osteoarthritis are effective only in treating symptoms, and none has been shown to be able to change the course of the disease and improve the condition of the cartilage. The new drugs being developed to treat inflammation, cartilage damage, and arthritis have numerous side effects. Recently, the most widely used nonsteroidal anti-inflammatory drugs—the COX-2 inhibitors—were taken off the market because of their dangerous side effects. Many drugs attack complex biochemical pathways present throughout the body and have damaging effects on organs other than the one they are targeting. The result is collateral damage in one organ system and benefit in another. The sad truth of modern medicine is that when symptoms of a disease are treated with a drug, patients develop collateral damage from the proper use of the drug, and then the new symptoms are diagnosed as a "new problem"—which is then treated using another drug. This is also encouraged by Medicare and other insurance companies, which reimburse physicians by assigning a code (called ICD-9) as a diagnosis for every patient encounter and symptom that develops. This encourages physicians to make a new diagnosis every time there is a change in a patient's condition, and a new drug is used to treat the "new" condition. In this manner a vicious cycle of **polypharmacy** is created, as is often the case with the multiple drugs taken by elderly patients. **Nutritional treatments** for osteoarthritis, on the other hand, have been shown to improve damaged cartilage in the joints and even arrest and reverse the disease process. Unfortunately, organized medicine has not adopted many of the basic discoveries made in the last ten to fifteen years that can help osteoarthritic patients.

Genetic research is unraveling many of the unique traits that predispose certain individuals to develop diseases. The new research I will be discussing shows that foods and other environmental chemicals that enter our bodies directly affect our genes, often predisposing us to diseases. A gene is a small segment of an individual's genetic code template, known as **DNA**. Each gene codes for a specific protein in the body that carries out a specific function. Genes code for specific proteins using a string of chemical compounds called *nucleotides*. There are four basic nucleotides that alternate along the gene that are known by the alphabet letters A (for adenine), G (for guanine), T (for thymine), and C (for cytosine). So a specific gene might look like the following: A-G-C-G-T. . . . The amazing thing is that while a gene is made up of thousands of **nucleotide base pairs**, a single base pair difference in the sequence is enough to predispose an individual to a particular disease. These base pair differences that spell the difference between health and disease are referred to as **single nucleotide polymorphisms (SNPs)**. There are about 10 million SNPs in the more than 3 billion nucleotide base pairs that make up human DNA.[5] The **human genome** refers to all the genes that comprise the human genetic code and that determine every characteristic that makes us who we are, from our hair and eye color to our predisposition to disease.

The genetic research that is unraveling the many SNPs that are important in determining our predisposition to disease is still in its infancy. As a matter of fact, this research is the new frontier of twenty-first-century medicine. Our genes are dynamic and are influenced by our environment, and it is SNP differences that cause some people to come down with illnesses when exposed to environmental toxins, while others are able to fight them off. For instance, we know that being overweight and having a diet high in unhealthy fats predisposes some people to heart disease. But not everyone who has a bad diet and is overweight will develop heart disease. This is because variations in each individual's genetic makeup determines the predisposition to develop certain diseases.[6] Future research on SNPs will allow us to treat patients in a more individualized and precise manner. I will be discussing in chapter 11 how certain SNPs influence a person's inflammatory status, making some individuals more likely to develop osteoarthritis. **Nutrigenetics** is a new field that examines how different nutrients interact with our genes to cause profound changes in our bodies. They often interact with our specific SNP variations to cause health or disease.

Many chronic degenerative diseases have environmental links, and emerging genetic technologies can be used to study these interactions more closely. Ongoing gene research is progressively unraveling these interactions, and new genetic engineering technologies hold great promise for curing the major diseases of the twenty-first century.

Osteoarthritis has a big impact on our society. It affects millions of Americans and costs the US economy more than $60 billion per year.[7] This disease is generally regarded by modern medicine as being caused by heredity, injuries to the joints from sports or accidents, and conditions causing abnormal stresses placed on cartilage, causing it to deteriorate. Abnormal stresses are placed on our joints as a result of excessive stress caused by being overweight, or obese, or from malalignment of the joint caused by previous injury to the bone or cartilage. I will show that the current epidemic of osteoarthritis is fueled by excessive inflammation as well as a dysfunctional metabolism in the body. In this book I will propose the **metabolic theory of osteoarthritis**, which is supported by extensive international scientific research. Our highly inflammatory high-sugar, high-fat diets cause genes to be turned on in our joint cartilage, causing the breakdown of that cartilage. "Suicide genes" are activated, and excessive **degrading substances** are generated in the cells of our joints. Under these conditions the cartilage cells become "plump" and begin breaking down the cartilage around them. In this inflammatory and dysfunctional state of altered metabolism, the joint's own cartilage cells become its worst enemies by producing substances that will break down cartilage. Osteoarthritis develops and the joint eventually deteriorates.

Physicians traditionally think osteoarthritis of large, weight-bearing joints such as hips and knees is caused by sports injuries and other conditions that produce abnormal stresses on joints. Being overweight definitely affects joint health. How does it do this? Is it simply the result of excessive pressure placed on joints by extra body weight? Why are obese, middle-aged women more prone to developing earlier and more severe onset osteoarthritis than their male counterparts? These are some of the questions I will explore. As we have discussed, those who are overweight are at a greater risk of developing damage

INTRO-1
METABOLIC THEORY OF OSTEOARTHRITIS

High-sugar
high-inflammatory
high-fat diet

Alters gene expression in cartilage cells and
turns on cartilage breakdown and
"suicide genes"

Cartilage cells become "plump" and manufacture
cartilage-degrading enzymes and chemical compounds

Osteoarthritic cartilage breakdown ensues

in their joints. For instance, it is known that obese men and women are prone to developing osteoarthritis at an earlier age and in higher severity than normal-weight adults. Recent studies have shown that being overweight is more detrimental to the knee joints of women than men. Why is this? I will delve into this subject more in chapter 10, which discusses hormones and osteoarthritis. It is important to realize that the hormonal state of the body plays a key role in the development of osteoarthritis. In obese women, complex biochemical and hormonal interactions occur close to the time of menopause that predispose them to joint damage and arthritis. These interactions are further influenced by poor nutrition, with high-sugar and high-fat diets, which generate increased inflammation and the formation of "**rust**" in the body. A high-sugar diet predisposes individuals to the formation of "**sugar-coated proteins**," which I will show are important actors in the development of osteoarthritis. The high levels of synthetic trans fats in an unhealthy diet lead to the increased inflammation that is so toxic to our joints.

The increased inflammation and "rusting" in our organs also lead to our hormones becoming unbalanced. **Hormonal imbalance** is a very common cause of poor health. All these detrimental states are at the root of the current epidemics of obesity, diabetes, and osteoarthritis, which are lowering the health and vitality of a great many people. Extra fat around the waist is referred to as **abdominal obesity**. Scientific research has shown that having an oversized waist is dangerous to one's health. The fat around the waist causes increased inflammation in the body by the production of inflammatory chemical messengers. These messengers trigger high levels of inflammation in the body by turning on genes in cells that produce degrading substances involved in the breakdown of organs such as joint cartilage. They also trigger genes to produce chemicals such as IL-1 that further lead to cartilage breakdown. Obese people are also predisposed to developing another condition that is on the rise in this country: diabetes. The presence of metabolic syndrome, with chronically elevated blood sugar levels and inflammatory fat around the waist, is a setup for damage to the joints.

People who are obese are often nutritionally starved! This may seem paradoxical, but because they often eat unhealthy foods with very low nutritional value, such as unhealthy saturated fats, trans fats, and high-sugar foods, they are deficient in healthy nutrients such as omega-3 fatty acids, vitamins, and minerals. This deficiency further increases inflammation in the body and also causes hormonal imbalances. Hormonal imbalances will be discussed in greater detail in chapter 10.

They include overproduction of the hormone **leptin**, as well as inability of cells to respond to insulin in cases of obesity and in people with diets high in sugar and unhealthy saturated fats and trans fats.

Americans consume diets with excessive sugar-containing foods, white bread, and pasta, which are quickly converted to sugar in the bloodstream. The overwhelming consumption of sugar, about 180 pounds per person per year, causes a chronic state of increased blood sugar in the body which leads to the development of **pre-diabetes**, also referred to as **insulin resistance**. When proteins in the blood are constantly bathed in a high-sugar environment, they become "sugar-coated" and form **advanced glycation endproducts (AGEs)**.[8] Recent research has found these AGEs to be involved in increasing the body's level of inflammation to dangerous heights and causing diseases ranging from heart disease to Alzheimer's. They are also involved in the "rusting" of our joints and the development of osteoarthritis. AGEs have been shown to cause cartilage cells to become "plump," thus initiating the process of cartilage breakdown.[9] "Plump" cartilage cells refers to the fact that cartilage cells exposed to increased circulating levels of AGEs begin to grow in size and start to overproduce cartilage-breakdown chemicals.

Progressive osteoarthritis, which is occurring more and more in younger patients, is a frustrating condition for physicians to treat. Other than the use of pain-relieving drugs and surgery, medicine offers very few treatment options. Diagnosing a patient in the early stages of osteoarthritis is not easy, because we currently do not have good tests to predict the development of osteoarthritis and catch it in its early stages. When a patient is eventually diagnosed with this disease, it is often far advanced, making it difficult to reverse the cartilage damage that has already occurred. When diagnosed late, it is hard to undo the chemical imbalances that were set in motion many years before. Early diagnosis will be aided by the new genetic technologies that look for **biomarkers**. Biomarkers are blood tests for certain substances in our blood, which are increased in the very early stages of the disease and can thus be used to predict development and progression of the disease. I will be discussing these technologies in chapter 18.

INTRO-2
THE MAJOR RISK FACTORS LEADING TO DAMAGE IN OSTEOARTHRITIS

1. Obesity

2. Metabolic syndrome

3. Chronically elevated blood sugar levels with insulin resistance

4. Excessive inflammation

5. Hormonal imbalance

By understanding the underlying chemical and hormonal imbalances that lead to the development of osteoarthritis, we can use nondrug methods to make cartilage cells healthier and decrease the destruction of cartilage. Using drugs to fight osteoarthritis is not a sound strategy. Drugs have many side effects by blocking key chemical reactions in the body. These side effects include undesirable reactions and disease development in a number of organs in the body including the heart, the gastrointestinal tract, and the kidneys. They also have never been shown to address the underlying causes of the disease, or to stop or reverse the disease itself—and steroids and nonsteroidal anti-inflammatory drugs, which are commonly used to treat arthritis, have been shown to actually *accelerate* the development of osteoarthritis with long-term use. The reason for this acceleration of the disease process is largely unknown. Using proper nutrition and nutritional supplements, we can promote cartilage-building and anti-inflammatory processes to fight the disease while avoiding the high cost and unwanted side effects of drugs.

Scientific research is helping us to learn much about the important mechanisms in our bodies that are involved in the development of osteoarthritis as well as the ones involved in maintaining cartilage health. By focusing on these mechanisms we can employ a more holistic approach to treating this disease. By "holistic," I mean the use of chemical substances (i.e., nutraceuticals) that support and enhance the function of cartilage cells as opposed to a pharmaceutical approach with the use of drugs that oppose chemical pathways by blocking chemical reactions. This blocking effect creates side effects in other organs such as the heart, stomach, liver, and kidneys.

Osteoarthritis and other degenerative diseases such as Alzheimer's represent a great medical challenge for this new millennium. They are comparable to the challenge faced in combating infectious diseases such as cholera and dysentery in the nineteenth century, and tuberculosis and polio in the early and mid-twentieth century. But the tools to treat degenerative diseases will be very different than the "magic bullet" drugs used by physicians in the last century. The major advances in the nineteenth century involved the discovery of bacteria as the cause of infectious diseases, the concept of sterility in surgery, and public health measures of clean water and sanitation. The twentieth century saw great advancements in surgical treatments and diagnostic methods. These advances have been critical to the success of modern medicine in fighting disease and saving lives. But the current medical **paradigm**—that is, the current way of treating diseases with drugs and surgery—is not going to provide the solution to the chronic degenerative diseases that are becoming more prevalent in the twenty-first century.

The current medical paradigm is flawed because it uses a double standard in dealing with new information. Useful basic scientific research in nutrition has not been incorporated into clinical practice. This double standard is a roadblock to doing large randomized clinical studies in nutraceuticals, because nutritional research is not as highly valued as drug research by the scientific community. The double standard is that modern medicine uses many treatments that have not been tested rigorously by double-blind, randomized clinical trials before they are offered to the public. For example, new advances in biotechnology involving implantable joint hardware, surgical equipment, and biologics are introduced into clinical practice all the time before they have been fully tested and validated by randomized, controlled trials. Drugs receive only limited testing by drug companies prior to being authorized for general use. They continue to be tested in longer-term studies only after they have been released for general consumption. It was during these longer-term studies that the side effects of Vioxx were detected, resulting in its being pulled from the market. This is not to criticize the past and present advances in medical biotechnology, but only to highlight that a bias exists when dealing with nutrition, nutraceuticals, and other holistic approaches that makes it more difficult to incorporate them into everyday practice. These are regarded somehow as "soft" and "less scientific" fields than drugs and surgery, partly because the average medical school curriculum spends very little class time educating doctors on nutrition and preventive care.

In this book I hope to show that a new way of looking at osteoarthritis and the research data that link its development to poor nutrition, dysfunctional metabolism, hormonal imbalance, and runaway inflammation is in order.

Part 1

IMPACT AND CAUSES OF OSTEOARTHRITIS

1

Cartilage and Its Role in Osteoarthritis

The major role of the cartilage in the joints is to act as the cushion that absorbs the stresses of walking, running, and other activities. It is useful to think of cartilage as being similar to the brakes in a car. When they are of proper thickness, the brake pads allow for smooth braking and stopping. As they become worn out, braking becomes harder, there is more grinding when the brakes are applied, and the car does not stop smoothly. Similarly, when joints with deteriorated cartilage are moved, there is grinding, popping, and a lack of smooth motion. This is very painful. But why do we lose the cartilage in our joints? Is this an inevitable part of growing older? The answer to the second question is "no!" Although osteoarthritis has traditionally occurred in older people, we are now seeing an epidemic of it in younger people as a result of their unhealthy diets. In answer to the first question, the loss of cartilage in the joints is a complex and poorly understood problem, which I will address in the following chapters. Osteoarthritis refers to the deterioration of cartilage in the joints and can be distinguished from other forms of arthritis, such as rheumatoid arthritis, which is an autoimmune disease in which the body attacks a number of other organs (lungs and heart) besides the joints. While much is known about autoimmune diseases, until recently the causes of osteoarthritis, other than those resulting from injuries, have been poorly understood.

Normal cartilage is able to absorb the stresses of everyday use of the joints and properly distribute them to the surrounding bone. Cartilage can be thought of as a snowcap covering a mountain: the bone is the mountain and the cartilage is the snowcap. A major part of cartilage is **collagen**, a protein that twists around itself in a helix and makes up the three-dimensional structure of cartilage. Collagen is the backbone of cartilage and forms the bulk of the "snow cap" described above. In this framework are dispersed the cells that build cartilage. Factories within the cells build the proteins that form cartilage, much like building a house from individual beams of wood. The genes in cartilage cells code for the proteins that are used to build collagen and the cartilage framework. The genes are the basic units of the "master plan" called the DNA, which contains the genetic information needed to create a human being. These cartilage cell genes are a major topic of this book. They are very sensitive to environmental signals such as the food we eat, the air we breathe, and other environmental conditions we come in contact with. When we eat the wrong types of foods, genes become activated in cells that code for proteins that break down the surrounding cartilage. Some of these genes are called "suicide genes"; they will be discussed in chapter 8.

In osteoarthritis, the cartilage that cushions our joints deteriorates. As it breaks down, the joint surface becomes irregular and does not glide smoothly. This causes the joint to become painful and swollen during movement, resulting in the typical stiffness and swelling seen in arthritis. When the cartilage is destroyed completely, a condition develops in which the two adjoining bones that make up the joint start grinding together (commonly referred to as *bone-on-bone*). This is very painful because bone, unlike cartilage, has many nerve endings and is able to perceive this abnormal contact. By this stage, however, it is too late to reverse the processes that set the whole deterioration in motion. Through proper nutrition and the use of key supplements and other nutrients, we can help preserve our joints and prevent the deterioration from occurring in the first place.

Cartilage is a complex three-dimensional structure made up of cartilage cells, water, aggrecan, and collagen proteins.[1]

Proteoglycans form the basic subunits of cartilage that bind to and interact with collagen to form the 3-D cushion of our joints. Collagen is not found only in cartilage; it is also present in many other places including the ears, nose, and blood vessels. It is an important component of the structure of the body. It is a unique structure in that it does not have the ability to effectively clear waste and ward off disease.[2] Cartilage is bathed in a fluid called **synovial fluid**, which delivers most of the nutrients to the cartilage cells. This is because cartilage does not have good blood flow, which is necessary to bring in oxygen and nutrients. It also has a poor lymphatic flow, which makes it inefficient in removing waste products that can accumulate in the cells. These characteristics create a perfect environment for the accumulation of toxins. **Aggrecan** is a major protein component of the cartilage framework whose normal function is critical to cartilage's ability to withstand the load of daily activities. Joints also contain fat, which is an important actor in osteoarthritis and will be explained more in chapter 10.

ANATOMY OF A CARTILAGE CELL

The cartilage cell is no different than heart cells, stomach cells, or any other cells in the body. A cell is the basic unit of life, surrounded by a wall, called the **cell membrane**, which separates it from the outside environment. Inside the cartilage cell, all the instructions needed to build a human being are found in the DNA, which is located in a central compartment of the cell called the **nucleus**. While every cell in the body has all the DNA needed to build a whole person, only a certain portion of the DNA is active in a given cell, depending on what type of cell it is. These DNA instructions are coded for by individual sections of the DNA called genes. Each gene codes for a unique protein, such as the collagen that forms the framework of cartilage.

The part of the cell outside the nucleus, called the **cytoplasm**, contains the chemical factories that decode the messages sent by the genes to form the proteins necessary to sustain life. These chemical factories, called the **mitochondria**, play a major role in the development of osteoarthritis. The mitochondria take the nutrients that are absorbed by the cells from the bloodstream and use them to generate a unique substance known as **adenosine triphosphate (ATP)**. All the food one eats is ultimately converted to ATP, which is the chemical cells use to power all their activities and to grow and regenerate. ATP acts as the energy currency of the cell, in the same way that money is the currency used to conduct our daily business affairs. In the process of creating energy from food, mitochondria create a by-product known as **oxygen free radicals** (cell smog).[3] This is analogous to the smog that comes out of the tailpipe of a car as gasoline is burned to move the car. These oxygen free radicals damage cartilage cells if they are allowed to accumulate. The body has unique chemical pathways to process and neutralize this cell smog (which includes the compound nitric oxide), but when one's nutrition is poor, these chemical-detoxifying pathways do not work properly, leading to the accumulation of toxic smog inside the cell.[4] This is deadly for the cell: its own waste products accumulate, poisoning and eventually killing it. In osteoarthritis, toxic waste products accumulate in cartilage cells, leading to the destruction of our cartilage. This occurs because the wrong types of genes are turned on in arthritic cartilage. The research outlined in this book points to poor nutrition as an important cause of this malfunction of the cartilage cell. It also points to nutritional strategies as important tools for the treatment and prevention of osteoarthritis. *Proper nutrition optimizes the function of the mitochondria, keeps the "right" genes turned on, and prevents the accumulation of toxic oxygen free radicals in our cartilage cells.*

CARTILAGE IS UNIQUELY SUSCEPTIBLE TO DAMAGE BY ENVIRONMENTAL TOXINS AND POOR DIETS

The cartilage found in our joints is a unique organ in that it lacks the normal blood flow, the rich nerve endings, and the lymphatic flow that is found in most of our other organs. This means cartilage is slow to heal when damaged because inadequate blood flow does not bring nutrients and other reinforcements necessary to rebuild and regenerate. The lymphatic system filters waste and carries it away to be disposed by the kidneys or colon. Because cartilage has poor lymphatic flow, it is prone in accumulating waste products and other toxins that circulate in the bloodstream. The toxins are stored in cartilage, and because of its poor nerve supply, extensive damage can occur in cartilage without any symptoms of pain and dysfunction. This is a dangerous set of circumstances that leads to the late detection of osteoarthritis by both patients and their doctors. These chemical characteristics of cartilage make it ideal for the development of degenerative disease such as osteoarthritis.

The body's hormonal state also has a direct effect on joint health. Our nutritional state, hormonal state, and overall health are connected at the chemical level. If we eat foods high in toxic trans fats, saturated fats, and sugar and white flour, as well as other unhealthy chemicals, our hormones, produced by such organs as our thyroid gland, start to malfunction. **Hormones** produce chemical signals that influence the proper functioning of cartilage cells and many other cells in the body. For example, when large amounts of unhealthy saturated and trans fats are consumed, cells start producing increased amounts of unhealthy compounds called **prostaglandins**. There are "good" and "bad" prostaglandins, but unhealthy diets overproduce the bad ones. Prostaglandins are the chemical compounds responsible for increasing inflammation in the body. When these prostaglandins are formed excessively, they contribute to an unhealthy joint environment, which leads to cartilage breakdown in osteoarthritis. These unhealthy

FIGURE 1-1
INFLAMMATORY AND DEGRADING CYCLE OF
OSTEOARTHRITIC CARTILAGE BREAKDOWN

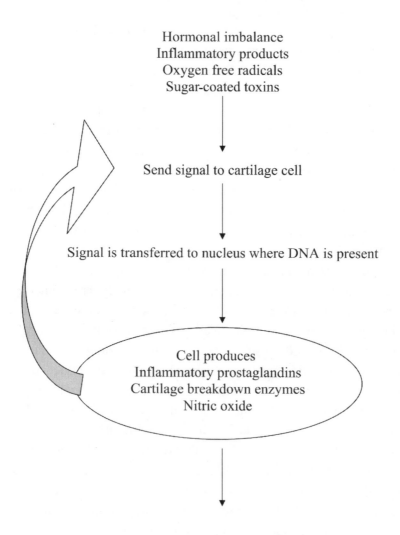

Hormonal imbalance
Inflammatory products
Oxygen free radicals
Sugar-coated toxins

Send signal to cartilage cell

Signal is transferred to nucleus where DNA is present

Cell produces
Inflammatory prostaglandins
Cartilage breakdown enzymes
Nitric oxide

These cell-derived inflammatory chemicals go on to break down cartilage prostaglandins are overly produced by the fat cells in the oversized waists (i.e., abdominal obesity) of obese people.

Our genes interact with the environment around us, and they are highly adaptable to the surrounding environment of each person.[5] In osteoarthritis, certain genes are turned off and others become overactive, leading to the development of this disease.[6] New research has shown that diet can control the expressions of genes.[7] An unhealthy diet can trigger genes that break down cartilage and lead to the development of osteoarthritis. Nutrition is very powerful in determining which genes are turned on and how they function. Each individual has a unique genetic makeup. It is interesting to note that the DNA makeup of human beings is 99.99 percent identical. It is the 0.01 percent difference that is important in coding for the individual characteristics that make each of us unique from one another. This 0.01 percent difference in our genes is what gives each individual a predisposition to certain diseases. Our genetic predisposition for disease—such as the development of osteoarthritis—runs in our family. What is important to realize, though, is that this predisposition is not etched in stone. We are not destined to always develop the same diseases our parents and grandparents had. Our environment, including the food we eat and the chemicals we come in contact with, influences the expression of these genes.

Cartilage cell genes code for three important substances involved in the development of osteoarthritis. First there is the production of **cytokines**, which are chemical messengers that influence which genes are turned on.[8] Second, cartilage produces **proteases**, which are proteins that break down and remove old cartilage as it becomes damaged over time.[9] This is part of the body's normal "housekeeping," but in the case of osteoarthritis, proteases are overproduced and damage healthy cartilage.[10] As noted earlier, DNA is made of short segments called genes. Each gene codes for a specific protein that has a distinct function in the cell. Proteases are normally produced in small amounts and function to break down old, worn-out cartilage as it is replaced by new cartilage. As we know, the body constantly replenishes our tissues with new ones—for instance, old skin flakes off as new skin forms. In this way, the body constantly regenerates itself. The problem in osteoarthritis is that these breakdown processes overwhelm the rebuilding processes: cartilage is broken down more quickly than the body is able to make new cartilage, resulting in an overall negative balance in the amount of cartilage remaining and the development of osteoarthritis. This occurs because increased oxidative damage and free radical production turns on genes that overproduce the proteases that break down cartilage. Thus, the whole delicate balance of new cartilage production and old cartilage removal is disrupted. Proteases are part of a class of compounds in the body also known **enzymes**. An enzyme is a protein coded for by a single gene that carries out some important chemical reaction in the cell. A third, very important substance is **nitric oxide (NO)**, a toxic agent for our joints that accumulates in joint cartilage as a result of poor nutrition. These three chemical, cytokines, proteases, and NO, are at the heart of the development of osteoarthritis.

Poor nutrition leads to the activation of "cartilage breakdown genes" and the suppression of "cartilage formation genes." In contrast, a healthy diet and the use of nutritional supplements that have been shown to support cartilage health can turn on genes that maintain the proper health of cartilage. Nutritional supplements are an important adjunct to a healthy diet and can be used to keep our joints healthy and to combat osteoarthritis. I will be discussing these in great detail in chapters 15 and 16, but some important ones include glucosamine; chondroitin; SAMe; **EPA** and **DHA** omega-3 fats found in fish oils; vitamins B, C, D, and E; alpha lipoic acid; and coenzyme Q10.

CARTILAGE IS SUSCEPTIBLE TO DAMAGE FROM ENVIRONMENTAL TOXINS

As mentioned earlier, cartilage is a tissue that has poor blood supply. This prevents cartilage from healing well after injuries, and also makes it unable to ward off disease or to neutralize well toxins that enter the joint.[11] In the case of osteoarthritis, as the three-dimensional cartilage structure becomes fragmented and dysfunctional, it becomes even more difficult for the proper nutrients to reach the cells. A cartilage-destroying cycle is thus propagated in the joint.[12] Interestingly, some of the most common drugs used to treat osteoarthritis, such as Indocin and aspirin, have been found by researchers to significantly decrease the production of the 3-D framework of cartilage known as the ECM or extracellular matrix. Please see chapter 12 for a more in-depth discussion.

One clinical research study in which 105 patients with osteoarthritis of the hip were given either Indocin or another anti-inflammatory drug, Azapropazone,[13] found that the Indocin group showed a more rapid loss of joint space and had a lower concentration of the beneficial prostaglandins in their joint fluid that increase the blood flow and blood supply of the organ. Loss of joint space is an indication of worsening of the arthritis condition. The decrease of prostaglandins in the joint fluid, which are needed to allow for adequate blood flow to the joint, can inhibit nutrients and oxygen from getting to the joint bone and other joint structures, such as the nourishing and lubricating layer that covers the joints, called the syovium.

In another study, researchers showed that **salicylates**, the chemicals referred to as aspirin accelerated artilage destruction and damage in animals with osteoarthritis.[14] Other researchers have shown that certain nonsteroidal anti-inflammatory drugs exacerbate osteoarthritis by inhibiting prostaglandin synthesis.[15] These studies seem to indicate that certain anti-inflammatory drugs accelerate the progression of osteoarthritis by reducing the manufacturing of important chemicals that increase the blood flow to joints. Presumably the prostaglandins blocked are those responsible for allowing adequate nutrients and oxygen to reach the joint.[16]

As stated previously, the joint cartilage sits on the bone much like snowcaps that cover mountain peaks. The ends of the two long bones that form a joint are called **subchondral bone**. For example, in the case of the knee, it is formed by thighbone, called the *femur*, and the shin bone, called the *tibia*. The end of each bone is capped by a thick layer of joint cartilage. This subchondral bone also plays an important role in the development of osteoarthritis. Early in the course of the disease, subchondral bone thickens and shows increased chemical activity. In the later stages of the disease, the bone actually starts to fragment as its fibers become narrower and weaker. As bone weakens it starts to deform. This is the reason people with knee arthritis develop bowlegs or knock-knees as the disease becomes more advanced.

CONCLUSIONS

1. Osteoarthritis is fueled by the turning on of genes that lead to cartilage damage and breakdown.
2. Poor diets high in sugar and fat, and low in vitamins and minerals, cause increased inflammation by the increased production of unhealthy prostaglandins, and "rusting" within the cartilage.
3. This poor nutrition changes the behavior and expression of important cartilage genes.
4. Cartilage-destructive genes are turned on, leading to the production of inflammatory prostaglandins that lead to cartilage breakdown and osteoarthritis.
5. Poor nutrition and obesity lead to increased "rusting" in the cartilage cells, which damages the cartilage. This is similar to the way metal rusts when exposed to water and oxygen for a long period of time.
6. In obese individuals, fat cells become chemical "time bombs." These fat cells produce inflammatory substances and destructive chemical messengers that turn on genes that lead to cartilage breakdown. This is why maintaining a healthy weight is important in preventing degenerative diseases such as osteoarthritis.

2
What Is Insulin Resistance?

CAUSES OF INSULIN RESISTANCE

The modern American diet is filled with junk food, sodas, pasta, breads, and "empty-calorie" foods. When we eat such a diet, our blood sugar becomes chronically elevated. Our bodies try to clear the sugar from the blood by picking it up and storing it in organs such as the muscles and the liver. The hormone the body uses to do this is called **insulin**, which is produced in the pancreas, a small but important organ that is positioned behind the stomach. In diabetes—a condition that has reached epidemic proportions in the United States—the pancreas does not produce enough insulin to process sugars, so diabetics must take insulin shots. If they do not take their insulin shots, sugar accumulates in the bloodstream. The presence of high levels of sugar in the blood is toxic to the body.[1] It leads to many of the diseases seen in diabetic patients, such as nerve damage (which can lead to amputation), blindness, kidney failure, and heart failure. Why is increased blood sugar so harmful to our bodies? It is because increased blood sugar leads to the formation of sugar-coated proteins called advanced glycation endproducts.[2]

When blood sugar accumulates in the blood as a result of excessive consumption of sugary foods and drinks, the body must produce increasing amounts of insulin to get rid of the sugar load. The problem is that as the pancreas produces more insulin, two bad things happen. The first is that the organs, which respond to insulin by removing sugar from the bloodstream, become unable to respond to the increasing amounts of insulin in the body, a condition known as insulin resistance.[3] The second is that the pancreas eventually gets "burned out" and stops producing insulin altogether. This is when **type 2 diabetes** develops. The occurrence of type 2 diabetes has reached epidemic levels in this country, and many experts believe that up to one-quarter of all children born in the year 2000 will eventually develop this disease if the current trends of poor nutrition and obesity continue.

A related problem is that someone who eats too many sugary foods feels hungry all the time. This is because both insulin and leptin, another important hormone I will discuss in chapter 10, are necessary to turn off our hunger switch in the brain. Insulin resistance has detrimental effects on the fat-produced hormone leptin, leading to the development of **leptin resistance**.[4] Leptin is produced by fat cells. Obese people who have insulin resistance have organs that are not listening to the signals of insulin (i.e., they are resistant to its effects). They have high blood sugar and also high insulin levels. Insulin resistance is thus referred to as pre-diabetes, as it predisposes to the development of diabetes. It also leads to increased leptin production by fat cells and also leptin resistance. *Excessive levels of these two hormones are important factors in the development of cartilage breakdown in the joints and the subsequent development of osteoarthritis.* The result is that people who eat high-sugar diets (also referred to as a high-carbohydrate diet) constantly feel hungry, even though they have consumed more than enough calories. This eventually leads them to become overweight or obese. The symptoms of insulin resistance include sugar cravings, fatigue, increased fat around the waist, high blood pressure, and feeling tired after eating a meal high in sugar.

FIGURE 2-1
HOW DO WE KNOW WE ARE INSULIN RESISTANT?

1. We crave sweets constantly.
2. We have a large waist, greater than 40 inches circumference in men and greater than 35 inches in women.
3. We are tired after eating a heavy carbohydrate meal.
4. We have low-energy levels throughout the day.
5. We have tiredness and low energy that is improved after eating a sugary snack or soft drink.

THE CHRONIC EATING OF HIGH-SUGAR FOODS CAUSES FAT CELLS TO BECOME INSULIN RESISTANT

When blood sugar levels become chronically elevated, fat cells start working against the body. They become "deaf" to insulin's messages, leading to the release of increased **fat** in the bloodstream, which increases blood cholesterol. This is because insulin-resistant fat cells do not function normally. They cannot process and store fat properly, which leads to increased blood cholesterol and **triglycerides**. The increased blood fat is also toxic to many organs,[5] and insulin-resistant fat cells generate **inflammatory cytokines** (or inflammatory messengers)[6] and release them into the bloodstream, increasing the overall inflammatory status of the body. Increased inflammation is the result of the production of inflammatory substances such as **interleukin-1 (IL-1)** and bad prostaglandins. These cause damage in our joints by triggering genes in cartilage cells that cause production of cartilage degrading substances and also by triggering "suicide genes." For a more detailed discussion, see chapter 8. The two important inflammatory cytokines involved in cartilage breakdown are **interleukin-6 (IL-6)** and **TNF-alpha**.

Thus eating a high-sugar diet not only causes weight gain, it also causes fat cells to become activated to produce inflammatory substances. *The "inflamed fat cells" found in obese people release inflammatory fat hormones that have been shown to have detrimental effects on our cartilage. This is the metabolic connection between obesity and osteoarthritis.*

The two important fat cell hormones I will be discussing are leptin and **adiponectin**. When one consumes an unhealthy diet and becomes overweight, the body produces increased amounts of leptin and decreased amounts of adiponectin. As I will discuss in chapter 10, both leptin[7] and adiponectin are involved in cartilage destruction. *The principle here is that hormonal imbalances produced by being overweight and having an unhealthy and inflammatory diet have detrimental effects on the body's organs, including the joints.*

HOW ELEVATED BLOOD SUGAR LEADS TO CARTILAGE BREAKDOWN

When liver and muscle cells are exposed to high circulating levels of blood sugar, they become insulin resistant and cannot absorb the sugar and clear it from the blood. This elevated blood sugar causes many proteins and fats in blood to become oxidized (rancid) and sugar coated.[8] The result of poor nutrition is the development of toxic and acidic advanced glycation endproducts. When AGEs accumulate in the bloodstream they produce a number of detrimental effects.[9] First, they cause increased inflammation by stimulating genes in cartilage cells to produce oxygen free radicals, TNF-alpha, and IL-6.[10] As discussed above, the latter two are chemical messengers that increase inflammation within cartilage, leading to its destruction. AGEs are also deposited in the cartilage by binding to collagen.[11] When AGEs bind to collagen, the three-dimensional backbone of cartilage, they weaken it, making it more prone to breaking down. AGEs are thus an important cause of osteoarthritic cartilage damage, and it is important to eat a diet low in refined sugar and sugar-generating carbohydrates—such as pastas, white bread, and other deserts—in order to prevent their occurrence.

THE RAGE RECEPTOR ON CARTILAGE CELLS BINDS TO ADVANCED GLYCATION ENDPRODUCTS

Recent research has shown that AGEs cause damage to cartilage by interacting with special chemicals called **RAGE receptors**, which are found on the cartilage cell membrane.[12] A receptor binds to a specific substance, usually a protein, located on the outside of a cell in a "lock-in-key" fashion. When the circulating substance on the outside of the cell (in this case, the sugar-coated proteins known as AGEs) binds to the cell receptor (in this case, RAGE) this causes a whole series of detrimental chemical reactions to occur that send the cartilage cell on a path of cell destruction.[13] The RAGE receptors transmit a signal across the cell membrane and into the nucleus, where the DNA is stored.[14] This activates genes that produce chemicals in the cell that lead to cartilage breakdown and the development of osteoarthritis.[15] The fascinating thing is that RAGE receptors are normally found on cartilage cells, but high sugar intake causes these receptors to become overproduced and stimulated to create toxic effects by turning on genes that destroy cartilage.

I have already noted that poor insulin function occurs as a result of unhealthy high-sugar diets. We can maintain proper insulin function in our bodies by eating a low-sugar, low-refined-carbohydrate diet. This means limiting our consumption of foods like pasta, bread, and sweets. Eating a diet rich in omega-3 fatty acids, found in coldwater fish such as mackerel, sardines, and salmon, as well as flax, improves insulin sensitivity and lowers blood sugar levels. Experiments with insulin-resistant rats have shown that fish oil, with its high content of **omega-3 fats**, reversed insulin resistance in these animals.[16] Proper insulin function can also be aided by aerobic exercise and by strength and resistance-training exercises. Taking the nutritional supplement **chromium picolinate** can also help regulate and maintain proper insulin levels.[17] This is because chromium picolinate works with insulin to lower sugar levels in the blood. Research has shown that when people who are insulin resistant are given this supplement, their insulin levels are lowered, blood sugar is lowered, cells become more sensitive to the effects of insulin, and also their cholesterol is lowered. Thus chromium picolinate is useful in preventing and in treating insulin resistance.

FIGURE 2-2
WHY IS INSULIN RESISTANCE SO DANGEROUS?

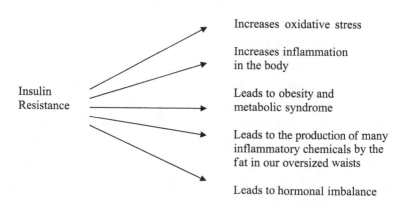

INSULIN RESISTANCE PROMOTES WEIGHT GAIN AND EVENTUAL OBESITY, AND LEADS TO INCREASED INFLAMMATION IN THE BODY

Chronic high intake of sugars leads to obesity. This may seem paradoxical, but foods high in sugar build more fat in the body than foods high in fat. The type of fat one has (for example, around the waist) is important in determining how much insulin resistance will develop and ultimately how inflamed the body becomes.[18] The more insulin resistance someone has, the more likely they are to progress to frank type 2 diabetes. The more inflammation present in the body, the higher the likelihood of developing chronic degenerative diseases such as osteoarthritis. People with more upper body fat around their waists, which is more common in men, are called "apple shaped" and are more prone to insulin resistance than those who are "pear-shaped"— most often women—with more body fat around the hips and thighs. We already know that obesity is bad for our health. The main reason for this is that obesity causes increased inflammation and subsequent illness in the body.[19] Fat around the waist is more inflammatory, and worse for our health than fat around our thighs. This is because fat cells in belly fat have been shown to produce more of the harmful chemical mediators such as IL-1 and bad prostaglandins than fat in the thighs.

Inflammation in the body can be measured by simple blood tests given in a doctor's office. Two such important blood tests are the measurement of two proteins in our blood called **C-reactive protein (CRP)** and **homocysteine**. Homocysteine has received a lot of attention recently because it has been shown to be as important as—or even more so than—cholesterol levels in predicting whether we will develop a heart attack. This is because heart disease is felt to be more than just related to elevated blood cholesterol levels attacking the heart vessel walls and causing blockages (i.e., **atherosclerosis**).[20] It is felt that inflammation, signaled by elevated homosysteine levels, present in these blood vessel cholesterol deposits is the real culprit in triggering heart attacks.

When C-reactive protein is greater than 1.0 and homocysteine is greater than 8.0, this is highly indicative of a dangerous level of inflammation in the body. These high levels predispose us to the development of diseases. Inflammation is beneficial to the body. By producing inflammatory chemicals at a site of injury, such as a cut in the skin or a broken bone, the body is able to heal. It is when inflammation is not associated with any injury or infection (thus we do not know we even have it), and it is also excessive and of long duration that it leads to disease in the body. For instance, it is known that people who do not properly brush their teeth and do not floss develop a chronic inflammatory disease of the gums known as periodontal disease. Pockets of bacteria accumulate in the gums that produce inflammatory chemicals that are released in the body. Chronic periodontal disease not only leads to tooth decay, but it is also linked to development of heart disease. This is due to the chronic (often silent until advanced stages) inflammation it causes. Nutritional habits play a major role in determining the inflammatory status in the body. A diet rich in healthful and colorful vegetables, high in **antioxidants**, low in sugar intake, and high in intake of omega-3 fats goes a long way in decreasing the inflammatory status of the body and in warding off the development of degenerative diseases.

CONCLUSIONS

1. Insulin resistance, a major cause of disease in the United States, is caused by obesity and the high sugar levels found in the standard American diet.
2. Fat cells, especially the ones around the waist, are very sensitive to the effects of insulin resistance, producing inflammatory chemicals and inflammatory hormones that cause the destruction of cartilage in the joints.
3. High blood sugar levels stimulate the production of toxic chemicals called AGEs.
4. Once formed, AGEs have many detrimental effects on our organs. They activate RAGE receptors on cartilage cells to start the cycle of cartilage breakdown and osteoarthritis development.

5. The activation of RAGE receptors has been implicated in a number of degenerative conditions, including Alzheimer's disease, and the development of hardening of our blood vessels, called atherosclerosis. This leads to stroke and heart disease. RAGE receptor activation is an important factor in the development and progression of osteoarthritis.

6. Insulin-resistant people tend to become overweight and eventually obese. Being overweight and being insulin resistant means that one has increased inflammation in the body. It also means that the cells "rust" and malfunction, causing disease. There is hope, though: Insulin resistance can be corrected through proper diet, which leads to a "natural" loss of excess pounds. Maintaining a healthy weight can prevent the degeneration of our organs.

3
What Is Oxidative Stress?

We all know that daily life, with all its responsibilities and obstacles, creates stress. Life is stressful! Stress occurs in the body in a number of ways, such as psychological stress when our job is threatened or our kids are not doing well in school, and physical stress from illness or injury. Here I want to concentrate on a special kind of stress called oxidative stress.

Oxidation refers to the chemical process in the body in which a compound combines with oxygen. This leads to "rusting," similar to what happens when a metal combines with oxygen. This damaging "rust" inside the cells is referred to as oxidative stress.

Oxidative stress occurs in our bodies when we consume unhealthy foods containing partially hydrogenated oils, refined sugars, white flour, and pasteurized juices.[1] Besides the formation of rust, consumption of these types of foods increases the acidity in the body and leads to **metabolic acidosis**. Acidity is measured in the body using the pH scale: a pH level lower than 7 is acidic, while a pH level greater than 7 is alkaline. A level of 7.0 is neutral and is neither acidic nor alkaline.

The pH level of our blood is tightly regulated to be about 7.4. The body functions better if the blood is alkaline rather than acidic. Diet is very important in determining the pH in the body. An unhealthy diet high in synthetic fats, sugars, and artificial ingredients leads to an overall acidic pH. A diet high in fruits, vegetables, and healthy omega-

3 fats leads to an overall alkaline pH. The consumption of unhealthy foods has reached record-high levels in the United States over the last twenty years. When the body has an overall acidic pH, this inhibits its self-repair processes and leads to increased oxidative stress. This leads to the breakdown of cartilage, similar to the way a piece of plastic dissolves in hydrochloric acid.

NITRIC OXIDE'S ROLE IN OSTEOARTHRITIS

Oxidative stress leads to the formation of **free radicals** in the cells.[2] Free radicals are unstable compounds that are highly reactive and damage the chemical machinery of the cell. An important free radical involved in the development of osteoarthritis is nitric oxide.[3] It is produced by the action of an enzyme called **iNOS** (see chapter 16 for further discussion of iNOS).

A useful analogy in understanding how nitric oxide is harmful is to think of it as similar to static interfering with the transmission of a radio signal. The static distorts the sound and makes the words unintelligible. Cells are the basic chemical factories in the body. Cells communicate with their outside environment through chemical messengers called **proteins**. Proteins in cells transmit signals that come to the cell from its outside environment and communicate them to the cell's command center, the nucleus. There, these signals activate genes in the DNA that tell the cell how to behave and what substances to manufacture. It is on this transmission of information that nitric oxide exerts its harmful effects.[4] By changing the chemical structure of proteins, it alters the signals in the cell and leads to the creation of "static" in the form of harmful chemicals called cytokines.

Nitric oxide is actively involved in damaging cartilage cells in osteoarthritis.[5] Together with other free radicals produced by oxidative stress, it activates genes that produce chemicals that deteriorate the joints, such as the cartilage breakdown enzyme **MMP-13**.[6]

Osteoarthritis is the breakdown of cartilage in the joints. This breakdown is fueled by our unbalanced and unhealthy diets. Unhealthy diet creates "rust" in our cartilage cells, causing them to malfunction and resulting in an acidic pH, which breaks down the cartilage. The cartilage breakdown occurs because this unhealthy environment turns on the wrong kind of genes in cartilage cells, which overproduce cartilage-degrading enzymes as well as the "suicide genes" that lead to cell death.[7] Research has shown that when human cartilage cells are placed in an environment of increased oxidative stress, they become dysfunctional.[8] These cells start overproducing degrading proteases that break down cartilage, they produce increased numbers of free radicals, energy production by their mitochondria becomes sluggish, and they exhibit damage to their DNA.[9] DNA damage is at the heart of the development of the degenerative diseases that are so rampant today. When DNA is damaged, the individual genes that form it are not properly expressed. Some are turned off, while others are stimulated to overproduce certain proteins. In osteoarthritis, specific genes called "suicide genes" are stimulated to produce proteins that lead to cartilage cell death. As the cartilage cells begin to die, they cannot maintain the tissue's three-dimensional structure, so the cartilage framework starts to unravel.

FREE RADICALS

In the cells, food absorbed from the bloodstream is converted to energy in the form of ATP. This process is performed by the mitochondria, the engines that drive the cells. In the process of using the energy created by the cell, they create toxic emissions in the form free radicals. This toxic exhaust is harmful for the cell and must be disposed by detoxification enzyme systems in the cell. If it is allowed to accumulate, the inside of the cell might look like the Los Angeles skyline on a smoggy day. When nutrition is lacking in the appropriate vitamins and minerals, the detox system malfunctions and free radicals accumulate.[10] In the joints, the result is cartilage breakdown and the development of osteoarthritis.

FIGURE 3-1
THE CULPRITS INVOLVED IN JOINT DAMAGE

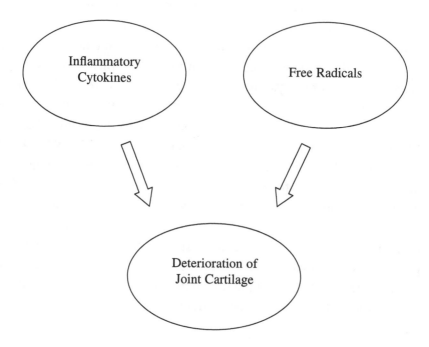

Vitamins and minerals are important because they act as helpers for the detox enzymes that take in free radicals and turn them into harmless substances.[11] Vitamins and minerals help to clean out the "sludge" that accumulates in the cells.[12] They help burn energy more efficiently, resulting in the production of less "smog."

Individuals have a different susceptibility to oxidative damage based on their genetic makeup.[13] This is because of small differences in the makeup of genes called single nucleotide polymorphisms.[14] Diet interacts with genetic makeup (in the form of SNPs present in key genes that code for inflammatory substances) to activate the genes that overproduce inflammatory and **oxidizing agents** in cells of susceptible individuals.[15] The lesson here is that a healthy diet keeps the correct types of genes—those that promote joint health—"turned on," while the wrong diet leads to the activation of genes that lead to inflammation and "rust" inside cells—and eventually cartilage cell death. This is why good food is good medicine.

FIGURE 3-2
RECAP ON VOCABULARY

Oxidative stress:	Internal body stress causing damage to our cells.
Metabolic acidosis:	High levels of acidity in the body.
Free radical:	A highly reactive compound that steals electrons from other compounds and damages our cells.
Nitric oxide:	A toxic agent to articular cartilage.
Proteins:	Messengers in the cells that communicate signals between the cell and the outside environment.
Nucleus:	The cell's command center.
Cytokines:	Chemical messengers that transmit signals to our cells. IL-1 and TNF-Alpha are well-known ones.
Mitochondria:	Chemical factories in cells that convert the food we eat to energy in the form of ATP.
Detoxification Enzyme Systems:	They normally clean up the toxic buildup inside cells. They malfunction when our diet is poor. This allows free radicals to accumulate and cause cartilage damage in our joints.
SNP:	Small genetic variations between people that predispose certain susceptible people to increased oxidative damage.

CONCLUSIONS

1. Increased oxidative stress and an acidic state in the body cause joint cartilage to break down, leading to the development of osteoarthritis.
2. Nitric oxide (NO) is an important free radical involved in damaging cartilage cells in osteoarthritis.
3. Oxidative damage to the joints is an important mechanism for the development of osteoarthritis.

4

Excess Inflammation Is a Setup for Disease in the Joints

CAUSES OF INCREASED INFLAMMATION IN THE BODY

Poor diet is a major cause of increased inflammation in the body.[1] Other causes of increased inflammation include injury, stress, infection, exposure to environmental toxins and allergens, sedentary lifestyle, increased waist size as a result of abdominal fat, elevated levels of the inflammatory protein homocysteine, and dysfunction of the mitochondria within the cells. Homocysteine is produced in the body, and in those who eat a diet low in essential B-complex vitamins, it tends to accumulate in the blood stream. Elevated homocysteine has a number of detrimental effects. It has been shown to inhibit the proper production and function of collagen, which is the important protein that forms the "backbone" of our joints. Homocysteine also participates in chemical reactions that lead to damage in blood vessel walls, which predispose to the development of atherosclerosis and heart disease. It also has been shown to be associated with increased fractures due to osteoporosis in the elderly. Increased homocysteine signals increased inflammation in the body. But, as discussed earlier, there are a number of things we can do to keep our inflammation levels in our bodies at an optimum level. It is important to remember that not all inflammation is bad. The body fights infections by mounting an inflammatory response, and increased inflammation in the body acts as a warning system to alert us when we are injured or when our organs are not functioning properly. The inflammatory response—with its production of inflammatory chemicals, pain, warmth, and swelling—is what is experienced when there is an injury or infection in the body. The inflammatory response is needed to heal the body. When pain is experienced somewhere in the body, it is the result of inflammation being present there. When one feels pain, one is alerted that there is something wrong in some part of the body. By developing inflammation at a site of injury, the body is able to recruit red blood cells, clotting factors, growth factors (chemicals that rebuild injured tissue), and nutrients that are used to heal and rebuild the injured area. The problem occurs when we develop excessive inflammation, which acts to damage our organs. This is when we are at risk of developing a chronic degenerative disease such as osteoarthritis.

BEING OVERWEIGHT AND OBESE IS INFLAMMATORY

When an individual becomes obese—as defined by having a **body mass index (BMI)** of greater than 30, then inflammation starts to rise in the body.[2] BMI is defined as one's weight in pounds multiplied by 703, then divided by height squared in inches. For instance, if you weigh 180 pounds and are six feet tall, you multiply 180 x 703 and then divide the product by 72 inches squared. Your answer is 126,540/5184, for a BMI of 24—within normal limits (25 or less is considered normal). A BMI above 30 characterizes obesity, which is associated with increased risk of developing heart disease, high blood pressure, diabetes, and osteoarthritis. Studies have shown that inflammatory blood chemicals such as IL-6 are increased in obese people compared to people of normal weight.[3] Furthermore, this increase in IL-6 levels found in obesity predicts the development of diabetes and future heart attacks—that is, the higher the IL-6 levels indicative of increased inflammation in the body, the higher the chance that a particular person with obesity will develop heart attack or diabetes in the future. These findings highlight how critical inflammation is in the body in triggering heart disease, diabetes, and osteoarthritis.

When we gain weight, our bodies start producing increasing levels of inflammation.[4] This occurs because our fat cells, predominantly those located around the waist, start to grow in size and become very chemically active. This chemical hyperactivity is not a good thing, because it causes fat cells to produce increasing levels of unhealthy fat hormones and inflammatory messengers (i.e., IL-1 and "bad" prostaglandins), which are then released into the bloodstream, with detrimental effects to the organs.[5] The organs involved include the joints (osteoarthritis), the heart (leading to heart attacks), and pancreas (insulin resistance and type 2 diabetes). These chemical compounds, such as IL-1 and bad prostaglandins, are able to "turn on" genes that cause cartilage breakdown in the joints and also trigger chemicals that damage vessel walls in the heart. Please reference chapter 8 for a more detailed discussion.

Inflammation is caused by excessive intake of inflammatory fats, such as saturated and trans fats, produced in an important pathway in the cells called the **arachidonic acid pathway**. When we consume large amounts of unhealthy saturated and trans fats, the arachidonic acid pathway in cells is activated to produce prostaglandins. Prostaglandins are the chemical compounds responsible for carrying out the inflammatory response in our bodies. These are the same compounds that are produced when we are injured or when we get sick. (Please see discussion above.)

While normal inflammatory responses can help the body to heal, a problem arises when the body produces excessive amounts of prostaglandins, which circulate in the organs and cause disease.

Inflammatory or "bad" prostaglandins work together with IL-1 and IL-6 to cause atherosclerosis (by increasing fat deposits on vessel walls), the development of insulin resistance, and the turning on of cartilage break down genes in the joints. The increased state of inflammation caused by being overweight and having a poor diet is not accompanied by the warning signs that accompany an injury. This is because the inflammation that occurs after an injury is accompanied by pain, swelling, or bleeding. The chronic inflammation produced by obesity, insulin resistance, and consuming an unhealthy diet is more of a "lower-level" inflammation that is unaccompanied by pain or swelling. It is thus most of the time hidden from our awareness. Because it is chronic, though, it has a cumulative effect, causing poor blood flow and organ breakdown. This is a big problem, because without those warning signs we are unaware that we have increased inflammation that can damage our organs or even kill us. People with increased inflammation have a higher risk of developing a heart attack, for instance. Until the moment the heart vessel becomes blocked and we experience the pain of the actual heart attack, we do not have a clue that our body is inflamed to dangerous levels. Inflammation in this case is hidden or silent, just as high blood pressure is silent. Most of the time we cannot feel we have dangerous levels of high blood pressure, and this is why it has been called the "silent killer." The same is true of the inflammation that develops in our bodies and threatens our health.

Inflammatory prostaglandins, which are the major cause of increased inflammation, can be decreased by eating a high omega-3 fat diet, avoiding excessive amounts of saturated animal fat found in red meat, and keeping the blood sugar level low.[6] Inflammation can also be decreased by eating a diet high in nuts and vegetables[7] and lowering the intake of whole milk, peanuts, caffeine, and excessive alcohol. Nuts are a good source of healthy fats (omega-3s and monounsaturated fats), vitamin E, and protein. For example, pistachios and macadamia nuts have high amounts of monounsaturated fats. Almonds are also a very good source of healthy fats. Walnuts contain the very healthy omega-3 fats. The problem with peanuts is that they can contain aflatoxin, which is a known carcinogen. Peanuts also do not contain the beneficial omega-3s as other nuts do. Caffeine increases cholesterol and blood pressure, and results in high blood sugar. These changes are linked to increased inflammation. Excessive alcohol causes liver damage and also leads to vitamin and mineral deficiencies, poor nutrition, and stomach problems, all of which increase inflammation. Whole milk has increased saturated fats, which have been described previously to increase inflammation in the body. Vegetables contain no excess sugar or unhealthy fats, which are known to increase inflammation. Furthermore, vegetables contain many antioxidants (substances that fight oxidative stress and thus decrease cell damage).

FIGURE 4-1
CAUSES OF INCREASED BODY INFLAMMATION

1. Eating a diet high in sugars, empty calories, and toxic trans fats
2. Psychological and physical stress
3. Infection
4. Environmental toxins
5. Sedentary lifestyle
6. Metabolic syndrome
7. Obesity
8. Mitochondrial dysfunction
9. Elevated blood levels of homocysteine
10. Insulin resistance

CONCLUSIONS

1. Inflammation is the result of a series of chemical reactions in the body that are fueled by the intake of unhealthy fats and excessive sugar.

2. Inflammation is a normal process in the body that acts to heal injuries and fight infection. It is carried out by substances called prostaglandins, which are generated in the arachidonic acid pathway in cells.

3. When we consume a diet high in unhealthy saturated fats, trans fats, and sugar, and low in omega-3 fats, our bodies produce excessive inflammation, which is internal and goes on undetected.

4. Fat cells found in fat around the waist become overactive in people who are overweight, producing fat hormones and chemical substances such as IL-1 and "bad" prostaglandins that wreak havoc on our joint cartilage.

5. A diet high in vegetables (with healthy amounts of antioxidants and plant nutrients), nuts, omega-3 fats, lean proteins, and a number of other active nutrients I will discuss in chapters 9 and 14 is important in lowering dangerously elevated levels of disease-causing inflammation.

5

What Is Metabolic Syndrome and How Is It Related to Osteoarthritis?

Metabolic syndrome is an epidemic that is sweeping the United States, but it is largely unknown by most people except for a handful of medical specialists. The word *syndrome* refers to the fact that it is not a single entity, but a group of unhealthy measurements of body fat content, blood cholesterol levels, elevated blood pressure, and increased blood sugar that predispose individuals to the development of disease.[1]

Metabolic syndrome is best defined as a condition in which a person has any three of the following five dangerous characteristics:

1. Increased abdominal fat, with a waist size greater than 40 inches in men and 35 inches in women.
2. Increased blood fat content, with triglycerides (unhealthy fats that accumulate in the bloodstream) greater than 150 mg/dl (milligrams per decileter of blood).

3. Decrease in the good fat in blood, **high-density lipoprotein (HDL)**, to less than 40 mg/dl in men and less than 50 mg/dl in women.
4. Increase in blood pressure to greater than or equal to 130/85 (remember that the top number of this ratio is the **systolic blood pressure** and the bottom number is the **diastolic blood pressure**).
5. Increased fasting blood sugar of greater than or equal to 110 mg/dl.[2] When we test our blood for sugar levels, we want to normally be fasting for at least eight hours. After a heavy meal our blood sugar will be elevated, but the body uses the hormone insulin to clear the sugar from the blood. When the blood shows a blood sugar concentration of greater than 110 mg/dl of blood, this means the body is not doing a good job clearing the blood sugar. This has detrimental effects as blood sugar remains elevated, causing damage to our organs.

The development of metabolic syndrome is not inevitable. There are a number of things we can do to correct the abnormalities noted above and help eliminate the occurrence of disease. Metabolic syndrome, with its associated obesity, high blood sugar levels, high cholesterol levels, and high blood pressure, is estimated to affect 47 million Americans![3] As discussed earlier, dangerously elevated levels of sugar and "bad" fats in our blood lead to increased inflammation, which, in turn, leads to the development of disease. Researchers have found that people with elevated fat in their blood as a result of excessive fat intake and abdominal obesity have metabolic syndrome.[4] These five factors associated with metabolic syndrome are important because medical researchers have discovered that people who have most or all of these conditions are more prone to develop diseases like type 2 diabetes, heart disease, stroke, and cancer. The initial chemical imbalance that occurs in the body predisposing us to to metabolic syndrome is the development of increased "rusting" in our cells. This is brought on by poor eating habits, a sedentary lifestyle with no aerobic exercise or muscle-strengthening exercises, and being overweight.[5] The increased "rusting" has detrimental effects on the energy-producing factories in cells, the mitochondria. Under these conditions, the mitochondria start to "leak" free radicals and other toxic substances, which causes the build up of "sludge" in organs such as our blood vessels walls and our joint cartilage.[6] This damages these organs, causing the development of disease.

Scientific research has looked at people who have low levels of vitamins and minerals in their bloodstream, and has shown that they are the ones most likely to exhibit metabolic syndrome and degenerative diseases.[7] These people also have increased inflammation in their bodies and are predisposed to hardening of the arteries (arteriosclerosis), which causes stroke and heart disease. The risk factors and unhealthy parameters that lead to metabolic syndrome are the same ones involved in the breakdown of cartilage in the joints and the development of osteoarthritis. **Articular cartilage** refers to the cartilage found in our joints. This is the cartilage that becomes damaged and eventually destroyed in osteoarthritis. People with metabolic syndrome are at increased risk of developing articular cartilage damage. Many osteoarthritic patients encountered in medical practice currently can be diagnosed as having metabolic syndrome. The mechanisms involved in this cartilage destruction will be detailed in chapters 7, 8, 10, and 11.

CONCLUSIONS

1. Metabolic syndrome is a major risk factor leading to the development of articular cartilage damage and the near-epidemic rates of osteoarthritis in the United States today.
2. Controlling the development of metabolic syndrome should be central to any dietary and medical treatment intervention for osteoarthritis.

FIGURE 5-1
DIAGNOSTIC CRITERIA FOR METABOLIC SYNDROME

Must have three out of the following:

1.   Waist size: > 40 inches for men
                      > 35 inches for women

2.   Increased blood triglycerides: > 150 mg/dl

3.   Decreased HDL fat: < 40 mg/dl for men
                             < 50 mg/dl for women

4.   Increased blood pressure: > 130/85 mmHg

5.   Increased fasting blood sugar: > 110 mg/dl

6

Obesity Is a Bad Player in the Degeneration of Our Joints

The incidence of obesity, defined as an excessive amount of body fat, has reached epidemic levels in the United States. According to statistics from the World Health Organization, 20 percent of American adults are obese.[1] Obesity is defined by using the BMI formula described in chapter 4. Please see figure 6-1 for more details. For optimum health, we should keep our BMI at 25 or less; a BMI greater than 30 indicates obesity. Obesity is more prevalent than it has ever been in history, with an estimated 60 million obese and 9 million severely obese people (defined as a BMI of greater than 40) in the United States.[2] That bag of potato chips or box of cookies is very hard to put down once you have started eating it! These unhealthy eating habits, combined with our overall inactivity due to lack of exercise and a reliance on the Internet and computers to run our lives from the comfort of our own couches, are changing the way Americans look and feel.

Our inflammatory and fattening diets, combined with the estimated fifty thousand man-made and often toxic chemicals—pesticides, cleaners, food additives—with which we come into contact every day cause changes in our genetic function. They turn on genes

FIGURE 6-1
BODY MASS INDEX (BMI)

BMI FORMULA

$$\text{BMI} = \frac{\text{weight (kilograms)}}{\text{height} \times \text{height (meters)}}$$

or

$$\frac{\text{weight (pounds)} \times 703}{\text{height} \times \text{height (inches)}}$$

RESULTS

BMI	Weight Status
19–24	Normal
25–29	Overweight
30–39	Obese
40–54	Extremely Obese

that lead to increased inflammation and joint deterioration in our bodies. While obesity and unhealthy diet are both risk factors for developing degenerative joint disease, proper nutrition positively affects our joints by decreasing the buildup of "rust" and decreasing the overall inflammation in our bodies.

According to government estimates, the rate of obesity among Medicare-aged Americans (ages sixty-two to sixty-five) has more than doubled in the last fifteen years.[3] Medicare spending has also doubled in the last fifteen years, and obesity-related illnesses such as heart disease, high blood pressure, and cancer account for a large portion of this spending.[4]

FIGURE 6-2
OUR DIET TALKS TO OUR GENES

Diet
Nutraceuticals
Vitamins/Minerals

↓

Interact with our genes

↓

Cause disease or health

THE FAT AROUND OUR WAISTS IS HIGHLY INFLAMMATORY

Obese people have large, active fat cells that produce a number of disease-causing chemical messengers and hormones.[5] Fat around the waist also attracts white blood cells, which are the cells responsible for fighting infection.[6] This in turn increases the amount of inflammation in the fat cells, which leads to the production of substances such as IL-1 and IL-6, which cause damage in other organs. Obesity is dangerous to our health because fat cells become dysfunctional in obese individuals, causing damage in organs such as joint cartilage by the release of these chemical messengers.[7]

Obese people are often also insulin resistant—that is, their cells have become insensitive to insulin because of its overproduction in the body resulting from chronically elevated blood sugar levels. As long as these individuals remain insulin resistant, they cannot lose weight. To burn off fat around the waist, the body needs to first be hormonally balanced. If hormonal imbalance exists, then the body is not able to burn fat and clear sugar from the bloodstream. This causes the fat to accumulate around our bellies and the sugar to accumulate excessively in the blood. The body must be sensitive to the action of insulin. This can be accomplished by avoiding those carbohydrates that are rapidly converted to sugar when eaten. These "bad carbs" are also known as **high glycemic index carbohydrates**, or *fast carbohydrates*, and include pastas, white breads, and sugary sodas.

FAT CELLS PRODUCE INFLAMMATORY HORMONES

When fat cells around the waist become enlarged, so does the waist. These fat cells are chemically very active, but not in a good way. They are responsible for producing inflammatory factors such as the inflammatory cytokines TNF-alpha and IL-6.[8] They also produce an important class of "fat hormones" called **adipocytokines**, including leptin and adiponectin, which will be described in greater detail in chapter 10. New research has shown that these play an important role in the cartilage damage that occurs in osteoarthritis. While these hormones are properly balanced in the fat cells of people of normal weight, in obese individuals they are out of balance, leading to inflammation, increased circulating fats and cholesterol in the bloodstream, and the perpetuation of insulin resistance, which eventually leads to diabetes. This is the chemical environment that leads to the development of osteoarthritis in younger people more than ever before. These chemicals are responsible for maintaining a state of insulin resistance that encourages the adding of more fat around the waist and in increasing our weight.[9] Forty years ago obesity was rare in the United States. Now we are seeing a new level of obesity called *extreme obesity*. People who are extremely obese—those with a BMI greater than 40— are often candidates for weight loss surgery, which has become very common. If we continue with our current dietary habits, what further problems can we look forward to?

WHY ARE TRANS FATS SO HARMFUL TO OUR BODIES?

Trans fats are toxic man-made fats that have been used in the last few decades to make many foods. These trans fats are vegetable oils that have been manufactured by the food industry in a chemical process known as **hydrogenation**. Vegetable oils are liquid, but by adding hydrogen to their structure, they become solid at room temperature. The reason this is done is to extend the shelf life of the foods to which they are added. An example of this is Crisco, which we all know that we can keep in our cupboards indefinitely. Trans fats are also popular because they are cheap to manufacture and they taste good. Examples of foods in which they are found include cookies, crackers, cakes, potato chips, some cereals, and baked goods.

Trans fats are not natural substances. This causes a problem when they are eaten, because the body does not recognize them as normal foods and cannot use them as energy or eliminate them from the body. They thus accumulate and cause harmful effects. They tend to accumulate on vessel walls, causing them to become hard and atherosclerotic. This leads to the development of heart disease. They also accumulate on the cell membranes, which are the outer coverings of cells in the body, and make these membranes stiff and unable to function properly. The cell membrane is critical in transmitting signals to the DNA of the cell as hormones and other chemicals come into contact with the cell. These trans fats coating the cell membrane prevent normal signals from getting through, resulting in disease. High-trans-fat diets have been linked to many diseases, such as cancer, obesity, diabetes. Trans fats also elevate the level of bad LDL fats in the blood and lower good HDL fats. High-trans-fat diets further increase inflammation in the body.

Omega-6 fats are necessary to the body's proper function. They cannot be manufactured in the body and are thus ingested in the food we eat. Omega-3 fats are also necessary to the body and must be obtained through the food we eat. These fats are essential to the proper functioning of organs and cell membranes. The problem arises in Western diets, which are high in omega-6 fats, obtained through eating red meats and cooking with oils such as sunflower and corn oil, and not high enough in emega-3 fats, which are found in flaxseed and cold-water fish such as salmon, sardines, and mackerel. This dangerously unbalanced omega-6 to omega-3 ratio results in heart disease, arthritis, and cancer. When we eat too many omega-6 fats, we stimulate our arachidonic acid pathway to produce more "unhealthy" prostaglandins and fewer "healthy" prostaglandins. This results in increased inflammation and increased clotting in the body, both of which are undesirable when excessive. Increased clotting causes heart attacks and strokes, and increased inflammation is linked to heart disease, arthritis, and cancer. Producing the "wrong" kind of prostaglandins leads to increased inflammation. Prostaglandins are messengers, much like hormones are, and they send signals to the cells in the body. They have important functions such as to control growth of cells, control the function and production of hormones, influence how much inflammation is in the body, and affect our blood vessels. A diet high in omega-6 fats activates the arachidonic acid pathway to form a prostaglandin known as E2. This causes increased inflammation in our joints by triggering cartilage cells to produce increased free radicals and other rust-producing substances which damage cartilage. A diet high in omega-3 fats decreases the production of the prostaglandin E2 and thus has beneficial effects in decreasing inflammation in our joints. "Healthy" prostaglandins have such effects as relaxing blood vessels (which helps blood circulation and lowers blood pressure) and have healthful effects on our immune system.

Eliminating the wrong types of fats from our diets can go a long way in preserving our joint cartilage. The goal is to increase consumption of omega-3 fats and decrease consumption of omega-6 fats. Eating the "wrong" types of fats increases the bad **low-density lipoprotein (LDL)** and triglycerides in our blood, which are known to lead to clogging of the arteries. We must also eliminate trans fats from our diet. The quickest way to eliminate trans fats from the diet is to stop eating prepackaged foods designed to last a long time on our kitchen shelves. High-trans-fat foods to be avoided include salad dressings, cake mixes, cookies, crackers, potato chips, certain cereals, French fries, and margarine. These foods need to be replaced by healthful foods including fruits such as cranberries, apples, strawberries, and tomatoes; vegetables such as broccoli, cabbage, and cauliflower; coldwater fish such as salmon, sardines, and mackerel; olive oil instead of margarine; nuts such as almonds and walnuts; flaxseed; and plant proteins such as soy and tofu.

ARTHRITIC PAIN AND THE ACID/ALKALINE BALANCE IN OUR DIETS

Arthritic pain is increased when the pH in our bodies is out of balance. Too much acidity, which is caused by unhealthy and toxic foods, increases the pain in our joints. In contrast, our joints respond well to a diet that alkalinizes our pH. An alkaline-producing diet is one that is rich in omega-3 fats, vitamin C, vitamin E, flaxseed oil, and B-complex vitamins, and high in plant antioxidants and plant proteins such as soy.

Impure foods loaded with preservatives, colorings, and trans fats cause the accumulation of acidic wastes in the body, which are then deposited in the joints. As you recall, our joints are poorly supplied by blood and lymphatic flow, and therefore have trouble clearing toxins that build up in them. They are thus prime targets for ongoing degeneration caused by free radical buildup triggered by unhealthy foods and toxins. Overeating is also inflammatory in that it increases the production of free radicals.

Our joints are damaged by increased inflammation, increased acidity, and increased "rusting" produced by free radicals, all of which are caused by excessively eating the wrong types of foods.

CONCLUSIONS

1. Obesity causes an inflammatory state in the body that leads to the development of degenerative diseases such as osteoarthritis.
2. We become obese when our cells stop responding to insulin and become resistant to its messages. This causes hormonal imbalances that lead to the increased storage of fat in the waist.
3. A diet balanced in omega-3 and omega-6 fats decreases inflammation and protects against the development of osteoarthritis.
4. High dietary intake of trans fats and unhealthy saturated fats leads to a chemical and hormonal imbalance in the body. This predisposes to the increased incidence of cancer, heart disease, type 2 diabetes, and stroke.
5. Enlarged fat cells in obese people turn on genes that produce hormones called "fat hormones" or adipocytokines. These play an important role in the destruction of cartilage in osteoarthritis.
6. Obesity poses a grave public health hazard and needs to be addressed urgently in order to combat the declining health status of our nation and the increased incidence of osteoarthritis.

7
Oxidative Stress and Osteoarthritis

THE ROLE OF MITOCHONDRIA IN OSTEOARTHRITIS

Mitochondria are very important chemical factories involved in the energy production of cells. In the process of generating the energy that fuels all the chemical reactions of the cell, the mitochondria generate inflammatory and other highly reactive compounds that lead to increased inflammation and cell damage. The mitochondrial factory is enclosed by a very specialized wall, called a membrane, which is made up of a high concentration of fat. This membrane helps the cell in its function of energy production. The type of fat present in the walls of the mitochondria determines how well they function in generating energy. If we consume a diet high in unhealthy fats, such as trans fats and saturated fats, the mitochondrial wall becomes very dense, causing it to be dysfunctional. It cannot transmit proper signals to the mitochondrion, similar to the way sound waves cannot penetrate a thick wall. When we eat a healthy diet high in **polyunsaturated fats** and omega-3 fats, the membrane wall becomes lighter and the outside

71

signals are better able to penetrate it. These lighter membranes are also more permeable to the uptake of important nutrients.

When the mitochondrial wall becomes dysfunctional as a result of our unhealthy habits and poor nutrition, metabolic imbalance and increased oxidative stress ensue. Nutritional supplements, such as **acetyl-L-carnitine (ALCAR)**, **coenzyme Q10**, and **alpha lipoic acid (ALA)**, which I will be discussing in more depth in chapter 16, help to maintain proper functioning of the mitochondria and their membrane walls.[1]

FIGURE 7-1
DANGEROUS HEALTH STATISTICS

- **20 percent of American adults are obese.**
- **Osteoarthritis affects 20 million Americans.**
- **25 percent of American adults have metabolic syndrome.**
- **50 percent of adults over age sixty have metabolic syndrome.**
- **A 673 percent increase in total joint replacements as a result of arthritis is expected in the next twenty-five years.**

FREE RADICALS AND MITOCHONDRIAL OXIDATIVE STRESS

As we have already discussed, oxidative stress is detrimental to cells.[2] This is analogous to living in a polluted city and inhaling dirty air, which is the cause of the high incidence of asthma in school-age children. Similar to high levels of ozone and smog in the atmosphere, oxidative stress is the generation and excess accumulation of free radicals produced when mitochondria convert the food we eat into energy. These excess reactive oxygen free radicals wreak havoc in our cells and organs,[3] causing leakage of the cell membrane and allowing toxic substances from the environment to enter our cells. This leads to the malfunctioning of the pathways inside the cells that transmit information to the nucleus. By disrupting important communications, free radicals cause unhealthy and damaging signals to be transmitted to our DNA in the nucleus. The DNA is the "brain" of our cells, containing the complete database that makes sure the cells function properly.

WE MUST SUPPORT OUR DETOX SYSTEMS TO STAY HEALTHY

The body is equipped with detoxifying systems that remove free radicals and other toxins as they accumulate in the cells.[4] These detox systems are nothing more than complex proteins coded for by individual genes in our DNA. For them to function properly, we must do our part by consuming a healthy diet containing proper amounts of vitamins, minerals, and other nutrients essential to good health. When the body is fed a diet filled with toxic trans fats, empty calories, and food additives such as dyes and preservatives, its detox system becomes overloaded and malfunctions. The result is accumulation of unhealthy "sludge" in our cells, which clogs the cellular machinery and depletes our energy. The detoxification system consists of three important enzymes found in cells, which are **superoxide dismutase**, **glutathione peroxidase**, and **catalase**. These enzymes convert toxic substances we eat or breathe into harmless chemicals that are then excreted through the urine or feces. When we eat unhealthy trans fats in large quantities and are exposed to a lot of environmental pollution, these enzymes have to work overtime to clear the body of these substances. In the process, they can become depleted and lead to the accumulation of toxins which then cause increased oxidative stress in the body.

In osteoarthritis, cartilage cells stop dividing and growing. In one experiment with diseased cartilage, researchers added vitamin C to the cells and found that their overall life span was increased and they became healthier.[5] The reversal of this oxidative stress environment by vitamin C is the reason it is referred to as an *antioxidant vitamin*—that is, it prevents the cellular aging and rusting that is the root cause of cell degeneration.

FIGURE 7-2
VITAMINS AND SUPPLEMENTS
THAT SUPPORT MITOCHONDRIA

Vitamins and supplements that are important in preventing the buildup of sludge in our cells and in decreasing mitochondrial free radical production include:

N-acetylcysteine (NAC)		1–2 g per day
B-complex vitamins		
	Thiamine (Vitamin B₁)	50–100 mg per day
	Riboflavin (Vitamin B₂)	50–100 mg per day
	Niacin	20 mg per day
	Vitamin B₆	50–100 mg per day
	Folic acid	400 mcg per day
	Vitamin B₁₂	25 mcg per day
Acetyl-L-carnitine		500–4,000 mg per day
Alpha lipoic acid		600 mg per day
Coenzyme Q10		100–600 mg per day
Vitamin C		1,000–2,000 mg per day
Glutathione		300–600 mg per day

These are important nutrients that support the detoxifying enzyme systems in our cells and are important supplements in the maintenance of optimum joint health and the fighting of osteroarthritis.

Another important experiment showed that oxidative stress damages the cell membrane, which protects the cell and functions to communicate with other cells.[6] This damage to the cell membrane in cartilage cells, produced by oxidizing and rusting agents, leads to the development of osteoarthritic cartilage breakdown.

OBESITY AND OXIDATIVE STRESS

Current research is showing that besides often having high blood pressure, chronically elevated blood sugar levels, and increased fat content, obese people also have a state of elevated inflammation[7] and increased oxidative stress[8] in their bodies. An optimum level of inflammation is important for proper functioning of the body, as discussed in chapter 4. It is when inflammation occurs chronically and at increased levels that it causes disease. Inflammation is carried out primarily by our white blood cells, which fight foreign invaders, and also by a complex series of chemical reactions that are critical to the normal healing process of the body. The most important causes of chronically increased and dangerous inflammation in the body are overeating and eating the wrong types of foods. The resulting increase in inflammation works together with the oxidative stress discussed in chapter 3 to lead to the formation of dangerous free radicals and nitric oxide in our joints.

FIGURE 7-3
CAUSES OF INCREASED BODY INFLAMMATION

- High-glycemic-load (sugar and complex carbohydrate) diet
- Stress (emotional and physical)
- Infection
- Environmental toxins
- Sedentary lifestyle
- High-trans-fat diet
- Metabolic syndrome
- Obesity
- Mitochondrial dysfunction
- Elevated blood levels of homocysteine
- Insulin resistance

The most dangerous type of fat is that found around the waist. This fat is more inflammatory than fat found around the thighs, and thus more dangerous to our health.[9] This is because when fat around the belly is excessive, its fat cells produce chemical messengers such as IL-1, IL-6, and leptin, which "turn on" genes in the body that increase cell damage. Thigh fat, on the other hand, does not exhibit these effects. When obesity around the waist occurs in combination with elevated blood pressure, elevated cholesterol, and elevated blood sugar, then a dangerous condition called metabolic syndrome is created.[10]

CONCLUSIONS

1. When we have an unhealthy diet, our cellular machinery malfunctions, food is converted to energy very inefficiently, and toxic substances accumulate in the body leading to increased "rusting" and acidity. This creates a toxic microenvironment in our joints that leads to the development of osteoarthritis and many other degenerative diseases, such as Alzheimer's and heart disease. Proper nutrition, including a number of nutritional supplements I will be detailing in chapter 16, helps cells and their mitochondria to function properly and prevent the development of disease.

2. The improper functioning of mitochondria as a result of increased cellular sludge, increased free radicals, and increased cellular acidity leads to degeneration and breakdown seen in osteoarthritic joints. The best way to prevent this is to consume a diet high in fruits, vegetables, healthy proteins, healthy omega-3 fats, and vitamins and minerals.

FIGURE 7-4
HOW CHRONICALLY ELEVATED BLOOD SUGAR
DAMAGES JOINT CARTILAGE

Elevated blood sugar

↓

Insulin resistance develops

↓

Liver and muscle cells cannot clear sugar by removing it from bloodstream

↓

Proteins in blood become glycated, or "sugar-coated," forming AGEs

↓

Osteoarthritic cartilage breakdown

FIGURE 7-5
THE MAKING OF AN
OSTEOARTHRITIC CARTILAGE CELL

DAMAGING STIMULI

sugar-coated proteins
hormonal imbalance
free radicals
inflammatory cytokines
broken cartilage fragments
environmental toxins

↓

BIND TO CARTILAGE CELL SURFACE RECEPTORS

↓

SIGNAL DNA IN CELL NUCLEUS

↓

ACTIVATES GENES THAT PRODUCE CARTILAGE-DEGRADING CHEMICALS

↓

CARTILAGE DESTRUCTION OCCURS

8

Inflammation and Osteoarthritis: A "Five-Alarm Fire" in Our Joints

OUR GENES INTERACT WITH THE ENVIRONMENT TO CAUSE DISEASE

When inflammation in the body is increased due to obesity, chronically elevated blood sugar levels, and poor diet, genes are turned on in our cartilage cells that produce inflammatory compounds such as interleukin-1 (IL-1).[1] These compounds are also produced by the highly inflamed fat cells found in fat around the waist.[2] Research has shown that IL-1 is an important inflammatory compound involved in the processes that damage joints.[3] Genetic research has isolated NALP3, the gene that codes for IL-1.[4] It has been found that different individuals have variations in the sequence that forms the gene code. As we have discussed previously, these changes are called single nucleotide polymorphisms. The word *nucleotide* refers to the alphabet-soup compounds that make up a gene. All genes are made up of four different nucleotides that are combined in long sequences and are coded using the letters A, T, G, and C. The substitution in one of the letters in a long sequence (for example, A-G-C-T-C-G-A-A-G-T-C-G . . .) with another letter is all that is needed to cause an SNP and change the function of the gene. Such an SNP change in the NALP3 gene creates a higher inflammatory response in that individual's body when exposed to inflammatory foods and other environmental toxins.[5] SNPs in key genes determine how individual people respond to foods and environmental toxins. These SNPs help to shape our genetic individuality and determine our predisposition to developing certain diseases.

Research has shown that unhealthy foods interact with the IL-1 family of genes and lead to increased inflammation, especially in these susceptible individuals. *This different gene functioning between individuals is at the core of why some people require larger amounts of vitamins and minerals in order to detoxify their bodies and stay healthy.*

INTERLEUKINS, TNF, AND INFLAMMATION: IL-1 CAUSES INFLAMMATION IN OSTEOARTHRITIS

Inflammation is a major factor in the development of osteoarthritis.[6] Inflammatory compounds such as IL-1 and TNF-alpha are increased in osteoarthritic cartilage compared to normal cartilage.[7] These inflammatory compounds are also referred to as cytokines. These cytokines start the breakdown of cartilage by disrupting the normal chemical makeup of the three-dimensional structure of cartilage.

IL-1 turns on cartilage breakdown genes.[8] When the production of IL-1 is increased, it also leads to activation of other chemicals that limit the ability of cartilage to self-repair. TNF-alpha further activates other chemicals in the cell, known as **chemical intermediates**, which trigger the "suicide genes" in cartilage cells, leading to cell death. These chemical intermediates, which transmit the inflammatory signals to the DNA located in the nucleus of the cell, are known as **NFkB** and **MAPK**. Recall that the nucleus is the storage compartment for the genes that make up our DNA. Thus NFkB and MAPK act to turn on genes in the DNA of cartilage cells that lead to osteoarthritis.

IL-1/IGF-1 IMBALANCE TRIGGERS CARTILAGE DAMAGE IN JOINTS

There are important chemical compounds in the body called the **growth factors**, which are small proteins that act like hormones in having regulatory functions. Hormones like growth factors regulate the multiple functions of the body and in the case of the sex hormones—estrogen and testosterone—they give the unique male and female characteristics in people.

One important growth factor in the proper maintenance of joints and in promoting joint health is **insulin growth factor-1 (IGF-1)**.[9] We have already discussed inflammatory compounds in the body called cytokines, such as IL-1. IGF-1 is also a cytokine, but it is an anti-inflammatory or "good" cytokine that counteracts the destructive joint effects of inflammatory cytokines. One of the reasons the incidence of osteoarthritis increases with increasing age is that IGF-1 levels in our bodies decrease as we get older. Studies have shown that approximately 50 percent of IGF-1 is lost in our joints between early adulthood and old age. Decreased IGF-1 levels inhibit the proper maintenance of cartilage and are associated with the predisposition to develop osteoarthritis.[10]

Experiments with osteoarthritic animals have shown that osteoarthritis can be successfully reversed by giving them a combination of IGF-1 and **pentosan polysulfate (PPS)**.[11] The IGF growth factors are very complex, and researchers are currently trying to unravel the ways this system interacts with other factors in the body to lead to the development of osteoarthritis.[12] Recent research has shown that when we develop metabolic syndrome and insulin resistance, IGF-1 levels are reduced, and this is detrimental to the health of our joint cartilage.

IL-1 and insulin growth factor-1 (IGF-1) have opposing functions in joint cartilage,[13] and when inflammation is increased in the body, IL-1 is overproduced and IGF-1 production is decreased,[14] leading to osteoarthritic damage.[15] IGF-1 normally antagonizes the effects of IL-1,[16] but the low IGF-1 levels found in osteoarthritis are inadequate to safeguard against the damaging effects of IL-1.

IL-1 and TNF-alpha are produced in increased levels by the body when inflammation is running rampant, and they are also overproduced by cartilage cells themselves. The local increased concentration of these cytokines acts to increase the production of **matrix metalloproteinases (MMPs)**, which are cartilage breakdown enzymes.[17] They do this by turning on the genes that code for these degrading enzymes.

FIGURE 8-1
INFLAMMATION AND OSTEOARTHRITIS PATHWAY

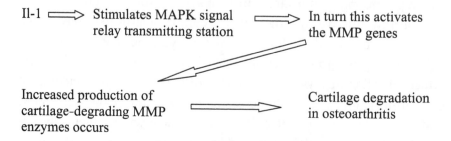

IL-1 produced as a result of increased inflammation causes the activation of MAPK, which increases the production of MMPs, which in turn start dismantling the cartilage framework.[18] This is an important mechanism in the process of cartilage degradation in osteoarthritis.

Research has shown that people with increased inflammation have increased blood levels of C-reactive protein (CRP).[19] CRP is an inflammatory protein that is increased when inflammation rises in the body. CRP elevation exerts its negative effects in part by increasing the concentration of the RAGE receptor.[20] As discussed earlier, RAGE is found on the surface of cartilage cells and is critical in propagating increased inflammation and in turning on cartilage genes that lead to osteoarthritic damage.

PPAR RECEPTORS BLUNT THE EFFECTS OF INFLAMMATION

Peroxisome proliferator-activated receptors (PPAR receptors) have the opposite effect to RAGE receptors. While RAGE increases inflammation, PPAR receptors are important in blunting the effects of inflammation in the body.[21] It is important, then, to help the PPAR receptors remain active and block the RAGE receptors by eating the right foods that fight inflammation.

Recent studies have identified **PPAR-gamma** receptors in human cartilage cells and have shown that PPAR-gamma stimulation is able to oppose the actions of IL-1.[22] A diet rich in anti-inflammatory omega-3 fats, found in fish and in the traditional **Mediterranean diet**, stimulates PPAR receptors. Omega-3 fats have other benefits as well: they lead to efficient sugar and fat utilization in the body. A diet rich in these omega-3s supports the function of PPAR receptors and decreases the harmful effects of IL-1. It also decreases the production of the harmful cytokine TNF-alpha, leads to increased sugar uptake by cells, and decreases insulin resistance. In this way, it reduces the formation of the toxic AGEs that are so harmful to cartilage. A diet rich in healthy omega-3 fats also decreases the incidence of obesity around the waist and the incidence of metabolic syndrome.

INSULIN RESISTANCE INCREASES INFLAMMATION IN THE BODY

When we consume an unhealthy diet high in sugar content, our pancreas increases insulin production. Insulin signals the body to clear the sugar from the blood by allowing the muscles and liver to remove it and store it as glycogen. Unfortunately, increased amounts of insulin eventually make muscle and liver cells "deaf" to the signal given by insulin. The result is that sugar accumulates in blood and insulin resistance, or pre-diabetes, develops. Chronically elevated blood sugar levels are toxic to the body because they cause the production of the sugar-coated AGEs.

Insulin resistance results in the chronic accumulation of increased sugar in our blood. Fat cells in our midsection that become insulin resistant start to grow in size and produce chemicals such as IL-1 and IL-6, which lead to to increased inflammation in the body. Insulin resistance causes AGEs to accumulate in the bloodstream, which in turn stimulate cartilage cells to produce oxygen free radicals, IL-6, and TNF-alpha. These cause increased inflammation in our joints.

INSULIN RESISTANCE IS CAUSED BY A DEFECTIVE GLUT-4 TRANSPORT SYSTEM

Increased inflammation in the body leads to the development of insulin resistance, which in turn perpetuates and increases the inflammatory status of the body. The release of IL-1, IL-6, and TNF-alpha in states of chronic inflammation lead to the **IRS-1** receptor to not work properly. When this receptor is not functioning normally, this disrupts the ability of cells to uptake blood sugar by decreasing the amount of GLUT-4 transport protein in the cell membrane needed to do this.

Insulin resistance is caused by the defective functioning of the **GLUT-4 transport system** of sugar uptake by liver and muscle cells.[23] In states of increased inflammation, with increased circulating levels of IL-1, IL-6, and TNF-alpha, the insulin receptor IRS-1 starts to malfunction.[24] This interferes with normal insulin signal transmission in cells, resulting in insulin resistance. The malfunctioning of the IRS-1 insulin receptor decreases the amount of GLUT-4 transport protein in the cell membrane.[25] Without this transport protein, cells cannot take up and clear blood sugar. The increased blood sugar (one of the hallmarks of metabolic syndrome) is toxic to the body.[26] Through its production of AGEs, it damages multiple organs, including the cartilage in our joints.

Insulin resistance is also caused when fat accumulates in cells as a result of obesity and excessive consumption of unhealthy fats.[27] Blood fat increases when excessive fat is released in the circulation by the dysfunctional "plump" fat cells found in the waist. When these fats are taken up by liver and muscle, they interfere with the GLUT-4 transport protein and result in insulin resistance.

INFLAMMATORY BLOOD CLOTS (ATHEROMAS) IN JOINT BONE CONTRIBUTE TO THE DEVELOPMENT OF OSTEOARTHRITIS

People with metabolic syndrome who have increased fat around their waists, increased blood fat with triglycerides greater than 150 mg/dl, and increased blood sugar levels are at risk for increased clotting in their vessels. This phenomenon, along with increased inflammation of the vessel walls, leads to atherosclerosis.[28] This is the "hardening" of the arteries by inflammatory fatty deposits that leads to the "clogging" of the arteries. This blocks blood flow, important nutrients, and oxygen from reaching the organs, leading to heart attacks and strokes.

Bone is a living tissue that is full of blood vessels, which penetrate the substance of the bone in order to deliver nutrients and oxygen to keep bone cells alive. An interesting finding is that the same clotting that occurs in the heart vessels (the *coronary arteries*) also occurs in bony blood vessels. When this occurs in the bone that makes up the joint, the plaques formed by inflammatory cells and fat deposits lead to sludge buildup on the vessel walls, which decreases the blood flow. This is the same atherosclerosis that blocks arteries in the heart. This decreased blood flow negatively affects both the joint bone and its overlying cartilage cushion. Decreased blood flow in the bone causes bone to start decaying and to lose its strength as the individual bone cells start to die from the lack of oxygen and nutrients being delivered to them. *The result is bone death and crumbling of bone, as well as decreased oxygenation and buildup of acidity and toxic wastes in the deep layers of cartilage that rest on this bone. Dissolved subchondral bone is a hallmark of osteoarthritic joints.*[29] This causes bone crumbling, which increases deformity when joint osteoarthritis is severe. Bone death and dissolution occurs by two mechanisms: increased inflammation, which leads to increased sludge buildup in the blood vessels that supply oxygen and nutrients to bone to keep it healthy and alive; and the overproduction of RAGE receptors which increases the breakdown of bone by osteoclasts.[30]

The hormone leptin, discussed in chapter 2, is important in the breakdown of bone. Leptin resistance promotes bone resorption (breakdown) by weakening and breaking down joint bone.[31] Leptin has been shown to be important in maintaining the OPG/RANKL system functioning well.[32] In leptin resistance, the system overproduces bone breakdown cells called **osteoclasts**, which break down bone faster than it can be manufactured. The result is bone loss around joints, which is a feature of osteoarthritis.

Leptin is important in regulating both osteoclasts and the bone-forming cells called **osteoblasts** to maintain delicate balance that keeps our bones strong and healthy.[33] Properly functioning leptin maintains normal bone density by inhibiting excessive bone breakdown by osteoclasts.[34] *The negative effects of leptin resistance on bone health combine with its negative effects on cartilage health to cause the deterioration of osteoarthritis.*

Recent MRI studies have found that in osteoarthritic joints, subchondral bone has decreased blood flow and is replaced in parts by weak scar tissue.[35] This weakening of the foundation on which cartilage rests accompanies—and may even precede—cartilage breakdown in osteoarthritis.[36] A number of studies have shown that joint bone in

FIGURE 8-2
ARTHRITIC JOINTS HAVE DISEASED
SUBCHONDRAL BONE

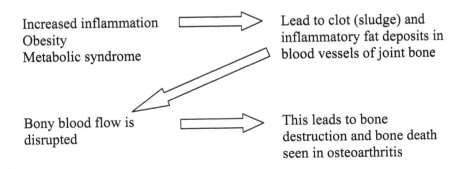

Increased inflammation
Obesity
Metabolic syndrome

Lead to clot (sludge) and
inflammatory fat deposits in
blood vessels of joint bone

Bony blood flow is
disrupted

This leads to bone
destruction and bone death
seen in osteoarthritis

people with osteoarthritis shows increased chemical activity, decreased bone density, and decreased stiffness.[37] The decreased bone density and decreased stiffness occur later in the disease process when enough bone cells have died and new bone is not manufactured at normal rates. This decreased bone density occurs only in the bone of the affected osteoarthritic joints. Osteoarthritis is different from **osteoporosis**, which is a generalized bone loss affecting all the bones in the body and develops usually in postmenopausal women as a result of decreased estrogen.

Increased body inflammation negatively affects both the cartilage and the bone in osteoarthritic joints. A link exists between atherosclerosis and the development of osteoarthritis. IL-1, which is increased when inflammation is at high levels, is responsible for triggering the deposits of inflammatory cells and fat on bone blood vessel walls. These deposits decrease normal blood flow in bone, leading to areas of bone death and the collapse of bone seen in osteoarthritis.

FIGURE 8-3
OSTEOARTHRITIS IS LINKED TO HIGH BLOOD FAT CONTENT

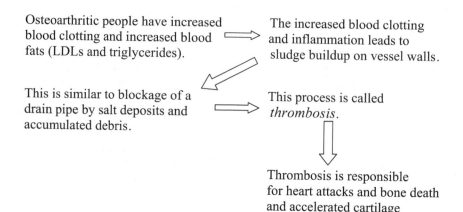

Osteoarthritic people have increased blood clotting and increased blood fats (LDLs and triglycerides). ⟹ The increased blood clotting and inflammation leads to sludge buildup on vessel walls.

This is similar to blockage of a drain pipe by salt deposits and accumulated debris. ⟹ This process is called *thrombosis.*

Thrombosis is responsible for heart attacks and bone death and accelerated cartilage deterioration in osteoarthritis.

OPG/RANKL BALANCE IS ALTERED IN OSTEOARTHRITIS

The **OPG/RANKL system** is an important "housekeeping" engine in our bones. Its job is to maintain normal bone density by regulating the balance of bone building and bone breakdown.[38] RANKL is a member of the TNF family of compounds involved in initiating cartilage breakdown pathways in osteoarthritis. RANKL stimulates osteoclasts to breakdown bone; OPG, which is made by osteoblasts, acts to block the effects of RANKL. As discussed earlier, all the body's organs are replenished with new cells as they age. This is done with enzyme systems that break down old cells and allow for new ones to take their place. Without this process our bodies would age very quickly and we would die. The OPG/RANKL system allows for the continual replenishing of our bones and keeps them strong and healthy. The dynamic balance of this system though is disrupted in osteoarthritis.

The disruption of the OPG/RANKL system accompanies the destruction of bone that occurs as a result of decreased blood flow in bone. Disruption of the normal bone anatomy and health can be seen on a specialized type of x-ray called a *bone scan*. Scientists have shown that when an arthritic patient has a positive bone scan, this is accompanied by progressive osteoarthritis and worsening of the condition. A "positive" bone scan shows the disruption of the normal bone because the x-ray of the bone scan shows a "hotspot" where bony destruction is occurring. A "negative" bone scan means that there are no hotspots of increased bone destruction. In one study, people with osteoarthritis who had positive bone scans showed progressive joint space narrowing much earlier than patients who had a negative bone scan. MRI scans of people with osteoarthritis show scarring and areas of bone death in the bone marrow (the inner portion of the long bones that make up our joints). Both are effects of decreased blood flow and a dysfunctional OPG/RANKL enzyme system. When bone starts to deteriorate, it triggers the inflammatory response as the body sends chemical messengers to the area to attempt to repair it. In this case, of course, the body is not able to repair the damage.

OSTEOARTHRITIS IS LINKED TO HIGH BLOOD FAT CONTENT

Research has shown that people with osteoarthritis have an overall elevated blood fat content. They have elevated "bad" fats, such as LDL and triglycerides, as well as an increased tendency to clot easily. There is an association between increased blood fat content and osteoarthritis. There are two types of blood vessels that allow for blood flow to and from our organs: **arteries**, which carry oxygen and nutrients to the organs, and **veins**, which carry away waste products and carbon dioxide. Clotting in arteries has been shown to be an important factor in osteoarthritis. Clotting in veins as a result of increased blood fat levels is implicated in another disease of joints, called **avascular necrosis (AVN)**. In this condition, blood clots occur in important blood vessels that supply bone, and the bone starts to deteriorate and eventually dies. This causes an accelerated form of

arthritis in which, as the bone collapses, so does the overlying cartilage. This is seen especially in large, weight-bearing joints such as the
hip. This condition is an increasingly common cause of the need for
total hip replacements in middle-aged people. Elevated "bad" blood
fats, which are the result of a diet high in unhealthy amounts of
omega-6 and trans fats, lead to increased production of "unhealthy"
prostaglandins such as E2, which increase inflammation in the body.
(Please see discussion in chapter 6.)

THE COX PATHWAY OF INFLAMMATION

The arachidonic acid pathway is a very important set of chemical reactions by which inflammatory compounds such as prostaglandins,
leukotrienes, and **thromboxanes** are generated in the body.
Leukotrienes and thromboxanes, like the prostaglandin E2 (discussed
in chapter 6) are "unhealthy" prostaglandins and are produced when we
eat excessive amounts of omega-6 fats as opposed to omega-3 fats.
Prostaglandins are important factors in inflammatory damage in the
joints.[39] The prostaglandins that are harmful are produced in the arachidonic acid pathway through the action of an important inflammation-
producing enzyme, **COX-2**. The anti-inflammatories Vioxx and
Bextra, which were recently pulled off the market because of cardiac
side effects, are COX-2 inhibitors. They work by decreasing inflammation and decreasing the pain of osteoarthritis by blocking the COX-2
enzyme. Once formed, PGE2 increases the activity of other inflammatory compounds discussed previously, such as TNF-alpha. The Vioxx
story highlights the fact that we must concentrate on more "natural"
ways of blocking inflammation in the body, rather than on drugs that
can have serious side effects. By targeting important enzymes such as
COX-2 and blocking them in organs throughout the body, drugs lead to
unwanted collateral damage. These concepts will be further discussed
in chapter 12.

INFLAMMATION IS LINKED TO THE PRODUCTION OF CARTILAGE-DESTROYING AGEs

Inflammation in the body leads to an increased amount of "unhealthy" blood fats spilling into the bloodstream. These circulating fats interfere with the action of insulin and of its efforts to remove sugar from the blood.[40] Once food is broken down in the stomach and intestines, sugars from these foods are released into the bloodstream. If the liver and muscles cannot absorb the sugar, it accumulates in the blood.

Systemic inflammation and increased blood fat impairs the GLUT-4 receptor, which, as previously discussed, clears sugar from the blood.[41] The resultant chronic state of increased blood sugar leads to the formation of excessive rust-forming sugar-coated AGEs, which increase oxidative stress in the body and rusting in the joint cartilage. Furthermore, as previously discussed, excess sugar in the blood increases inflammation[42] and turns on genes that produce cartilage-degrading enzymes.

Thus, inflammation and increased sugar-coated proteins work together to stimulate the production of increased MMP enzymes in cartilage, which carry out the osteoarthritic cartilage breakdown.

LEUKOTRIENE B4 AND OTHER INFLAMMATORY PROSTAGLANDINS

In states of increased body inflammation, compounds called leukotrienes are produced through the activation of the **LOX enzyme** in the arachidonic acid pathway.[43] Leukotrienes are inflammatory prostaglandins whose production is increased because inflammation in the body increases the activity of the LOX enzyme. The LOX enzyme is activated to produce inflammatory prostaglandins when we eat a diet high in omega-6 fats and low in omega-3 fats.

Research with arthritic mice has shown that when the genes that are responsible for coding for **leukotriene LTB4** were blocked, the mice did not develop progressive arthritis.[44] LTB4 acts through the transmitting relay station NFkB to generate large numbers of oxygen free radicals. NFkB (nuclear factor KB), is a chemical compound in cells that, when an "unhealthy" prostaglandin such as LTB4 stimulates the cell, transmits this harmful signal to the DNA of the cell in the nucleus. These genes, which code for cartilage-breakdown proteases and free radicals, are turned on. NFkB is also responsible for attracting white blood cells into joints; this increases the inflammatory response. The white cells do not attack the body in osteoarthritis, but they do increase inflammation. NFkB further increases the synthesis of IL-1-beta, an inflammatory compound in osteoarthritic joints that is responsible for producing more cartilage destruction.

ANTI-INFLAMMATORY DRUGS:
THE EVIDENCE OF DETRIMENTAL EFFECTS
ON JOINT CARTILAGE

Anti-inflammatory drugs are widely used to control the pain of osteoarthritis. What is not widely known is that these drugs promote cartilage deterioration when used for long periods. They increase the synthesis of leukotriene LTB4 and IL-1-beta. As discussed earlier, anti-inflammatory drugs exert their positive pain-relieving action by blocking the COX enzyme in the arachidonic acid pathway. In doing so, they cause an unwanted shift of the arachidonic acid that is consumed in our unhealthy diets to be processed through the LOX pathway (a series of chemical reactions that involve the LOX enzyme, discussed above, and lead to the overproduction of "unhealthy" prostaglandins), leading to increased production of inflammatory LTB4.

Drugs can have a positive effect by blocking one pathway (COX) while also having negative effects by increasing the activity of another pathway (LOX). This is an example of the dual nature of drugs: While drugs can have benefits, they can also cause unwanted side effects. The benefits produced as well as the side effects created must be balanced for each patient and each condition in order to determine whether the drug is appropriate for the situation. One of the problems with drugs is that while the actions that benefit the body are often well understood, their potential dangerous side effects and toxicity are not known early on. This is why drugs released for general consumption are sometimes later pulled off the market. *The drawback of drugs is that they block specific pathways in an indiscriminate fashion across multiple organs in the body.* While they help one organ, they can potentially damage another. This is because the specific chemical reactions they block have multiple and often differing functions in different organs. Furthermore, there is a delicate balance in the body of the multiple chemical pathways that constitute our metabolism.

Researchers in Sweden have shown that nonsteroidal anti-inflammatory drugs—and specifically the newer COX-2 inhibitors—have detrimental effects on cartilage, bone, and tendon repair.[45] Nonsteroidals have also been shown to block the normal protein synthesis needed to maintain muscle mass. COX-2 inhibitors block prostaglandin synthesis, and because prostaglandins are essential for proper bone healing after a fracture, this has the effect of slowing the healing of fractures.

THE ARACHIDONIC ACID PATHWAY AND PROSTAGLANDINS

Prostaglandins—the fat compounds produced in the arachidonic acid pathway—play an important role in the development of osteoarthritis. An individual's diet determines whether a preponderance of "good" or "harmful" prostaglandins are produced.

Prostaglandins act as messengers in the body and are similar to hormones in that they influence the function of cells. The good prostaglandins, such as those produced by a diet high in omega-3 fats, stimulate anti-inflammatory pathways, while the harmful ones, such as ones produced by a diet high omega-6 fats, activate inflammatory ones. These inflammatory pathways trigger the increase in IL-6 and TNF-alpha cytokine production. These inflammatory compounds produced in inflammatory pathways, such as the LOX pathway, in turn initiate joint destruction in osteoarthritis. These inflammatory cytokines further act to trigger the development of pre-diabetes and help form more toxic sugar-coated proteins and oxygen free radicals, which also conspire to destroy joint cartilage.

Inflammatory prostaglandins are formed when excess arachidonic acid accumulates in the oversized waists of obese people and those with metabolic syndrome. Diets high in anti-inflammatory omega-3 fats positively affect inflammation by blocking the formation of arachidonic acid and the subsequent formation of inflammatory prostaglandins such as the leukotrienes.

INFLAMMATORY CYTOKINES ARE LOCALLY PRODUCED IN ARTHRITIS JOINTS

Inflammatory cytokines are produced in inflammatory fat cells both in the waist and in osteoarthritic joints. Research has shown that fat in the joints of arthritic patients produces increased amounts of these inflammatory cytokines, which are released into the joint fluid that bathes the cartilage.[46] There these inflammatory compounds, including TNF-alpha, **VEGF**, and IL-6, cause cartilage damage.

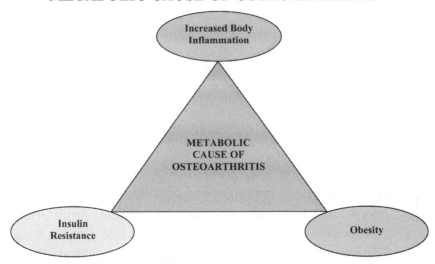

FIGURE 8-4
THE TERRIBLE TRIAD:
METABOLIC CAUSE OF OSTEOARTHRITIS

THE BENEFICIAL EFFECTS OF DIET ON INFLAMMATION

A number of studies have shown the positive effects of good nutrition on the inflammation status of our bodies.[47] Specifically, the Mediterranean diet, which is high in beneficial omega-3 fats, nuts, olive oil, and vegetables, has been studied in large populations and has been shown to decrease inflammation by lowering the levels of inflammatory compounds measured in the blood, such as CRP, IL-6, TNF-alpha, and homocysteine.[48] This diet also lowers blood clotting in the body, helping to preventing strokes, heart attacks, and also the clogging of bone blood vessels in the joints. The studies have also shown a dose-related effect of the Mediterranean diet in decreasing inflammation—that is, the people most adherent to the diet had a more significant reduction in inflammation in their bodies compared to those who were less adherent.[49]

Contrary to popular belief, scientific studies have shown that the

Mediterranean diet, which is a "high-fat" diet—approximately 30 percent fat—is better than a low-fat diet for preventing heart disease. The heart-protective effects of the Mediterranean diet[50] are related to its decrease in inflammation and its inclusion of healthy omega-3 fats and olive oil, which do not cause "unhealthful" prostaglandins to be produced.[51] The conclusion of large studies is that the Mediterranean diet prevents the development of new heart attacks better than a low-fat diet.[52] Thus, eating the Mediterranean diet produces fewer blood clotting events and lower incidence of atherosclerosis, which is also beneficial in maintaining good bone circulation in our joints and lessening the risk for osteoarthritis.

Long-term studies of patients on the Mediterranean diet versus those on low-fat diets showed that people on the Mediterranean diet had greater weight loss, lower CRP levels, decreased insulin resistance, decreased cholesterol and triglycerides, and decreased production of inflammatory cytokine compounds in the blood.[53] The Mediterranean diet is beneficial in improving metabolic syndrome, in lowering inflammation, and in decreasing the risk of blood vessel clotting.[54] People who eat a Mediterranean diet have decreased numbers of platelets in their blood and thus have decreased clotting propensity.[55] This lowered clotting decreases the risk of developing atherosclerosis and the formation of sludge on vessel walls that can cause heart attacks and bone deterioration in arthritic joints.

CONCLUSIONS

1. The development of insulin resistance leads to the formation of advanced glycation endproducts, which are key players in the stimulation of cartilage breakdown.
2. Inflammatory cytokines such as IL-1, TNF-alpha, and IL-6 are increased when our blood sugar levels are constantly elevated.
3. Inflammation is increased in insulin-resistant patients and during states of increased blood sugar.

FIGURE 8-5
MEDITERRANEAN DIET

Key foods that are part of the Mediterranean diet include:

1. Coldwater fish rich in omega-3 fats (salmon, mackerel, sardines)

2. Nuts (walnuts, almonds)

3. Olive oil (monounsaturated fat)

4. Fruits

5. Vegetables

6. Red wine

7. White meat (low in saturated fat)

8. Vegetable proteins (olives, beans, soy, nuts)

4. High sugar intake in our diet causes inflammation, which leads to disease in our bodies.
5. Metabolic syndrome and obesity lead to atherosclerosis, with increased inflammatory sludge deposited in blood vessels.
6. The sluggish blood flow resulting from atherosclerosis of bone blood vessels leads to damage in bone and to the bone death seen in osteoarthritis. The crumbling of bone results in disruption of cartilage, similar to a faultline eruption from an earthquake. The cartilage becomes ruptured and the fragmentation process is intensified.
7. People with increased blood fat content and increased blood clotting have an increased risk of developing osteoarthritis.
8. High blood sugar levels increase inflammation and increase the production of the compound arachidonic acid, which fuels

increased inflammation in the body. Arachidonic acid is found in excess amounts and stored in the fat cells of people with obesity.

9. Arachidonic acid leads to the formation of inflammatory prostaglandins and leukotrienes.

10. High blood sugar levels lead to an increase of AGEs in the blood, which in turn increase the production of rust-forming free radicals in the joints. NFkB is activated by the AGEs and "turns on" inflammatory genes in the joints.

11. High blood sugar levels lead to increased inflammation and are directly involved in activating pathways that lead to osteoarthritic cartilage damage.

12. A diet high in unhealthy fats leads to increased inflammation, increased incidence of metabolic syndrome, increased cardio-vascular disease, and increased blood clotting.

13. The classic Mediterranean diet can lower the incidence of the many chronic degenerative diseases plaguing us during the twenty-first century, and it is also the best diet for people suffering from osteoarthritis.

Part 2

NEW NUTRITIONAL RESEARCH AND OSTEOARTHRITIS

9

Omega-3s: The Good Fats That Quench the Fire of Inflammation

OMEGA-3S AND ARTICULAR CARTILAGE

A number of studies have been performed looking at the effects of the healthful omega-3 fats and osteoarthritis. Scientists have exposed osteoarthritic cartilage cells to omega-3 fats, which are taken up by the cells and have been shown to decrease the enzymes that carry out cartilage breakdown. Osteoarthritic cartilage cells overproduce a class of enzymes known as MMPs.[1] MMPs are normally produced by cartilage cells and are responsible for removing old cartilage as it ages and replacing it with new cartilage in our joints. This is part of the normal "housekeeping" function of the body, in which our organs are constantly renewed at the cellular level. But in the case of osteoarthritis, the genes that code for the MMP protease enzymes are overly stimulated, producing an excessive amount of these cartilage-degrading enzymes.[2] Experiments have shown that cartilage destruction was decreased in the presence of these healthful omega-3 fats.[3] This is because these fats are taken up by cells and are incorporated in the cell membrane. Cell membranes have a high content of fat in their structure, and when this fat is the right type they function well. (Please see chapter 6 for an in-depth discussion of "good" and "bad" fats.) The incorporation of omega-3s in cartilage cell membranes makes these cells healthier and sends signals to their DNA to decrease the production of inflammatory substances and cartilage-degrading enzymes. These studies highlight the powerful effects of nutrients such as omega-3s in altering **gene expression** and leading to healthier cartilage cells.[4]

Other studies have shown that omega-3 fatty acids, such as EPA (the beneficial omega-3 fatty acids found in salmon and other cold-water fish), are able to increase the **collagen synthesis** of cartilage cells.[5]

The conclusion of the many studies on the effects of omega-3 fats on cartilage is that diets supplemented with omega-3 fats have cartilage-protective and anti-inflammatory effects and are thus beneficial in the treatment of osteoarthritis. Omega-3 fats are thus important **nutraceuticals**. Nutraceuticals are nutritional substances with beneficial effects in treating and preventing disease. As an example of the importance of omega-3 fats, certain people with a single nucleotide polymorphism in a gene that produces the enzyme arachidonate 5-lipoxygenase have been shown by researchers to have increased inflammation in their bodies when eating a diet low in omega-3s. Because we do not have the ability to genetically test every individual for this particular SNP, it is recommended that everyone should strive to increase the amount of omega-3 fats in their diets. Omega-3 fatty acids can help decrease the inflammatory symptoms of osteoarthritis. Omega-3 dietary treatment of degenerative joint disease works by decreasing the production of harmful substances (inflammatory prostaglandins and MMPs) by directly blocking the genes that code for these substances and decreasing the overall inflammation in the body.

OMEGA-3 FATS ARE GOOD FOR BONE

The effects of omega-3s on bone have also been studied. As discussed earlier, a joint is made up of the ends of two adjoining bones that are covered by a white cap of cartilage cushion. The joint moves as these cartilage-covered subchondral bones glide past each other. Scientific studies have shown that omega-3s exert positive effects on bone. They have beneficial effects in decreasing the risk of development of osteoporosis, or weakening of bone.[6] Animal studies have shown that omega-3 fats increase the strength of bones, especially in estrogen-deficient postmenopausal animals.[7]

OMEGA-3S FIGHT INFLAMMATION

One of the major causes of increased inflammation is the consumption of unhealthy trans fats and excessive consumption of saturated fats found in red meats. Trans fats should be completely or nearly completely eliminated from the diet. In the case of saturated fats, they should be consumed significantly less than omega-3 fats. I would recommend eating chicken and salmon over red meat for the vast majority of the meals in which animal protein is consumed. When we increase the amount of omega-3s we eat, we reduce the fire of inflammation in our bodies. An important study of a group of 727 female nurses showed that intake of omega-3s lowered blood levels of inflammatory biomarkers such as ESR in these women.[8] Other studies have shown also that regular intake of omega-3s lowers inflammation in the body and improves overall health.[9] Even significantly overweight people who also have metabolic syndrome, when given a diet rich in omega-3 fats, showed a decrease in their overall inflammation and lessening of their metabolic syndrome state.[10] Diets rich in omega-3s help the body incorporate these healthful fats into the cell membrane rather than the inflammatory arachidonic acid fat.

OMEGA-3s STIMULATE PPAR RECEPTORS AND DECREASE INFLAMMATION

Recent research has shown that omega-3s are absorbed into the bloodstream and interact with specific cellular receptors called **PPAR-alpha** receptors. Receptors are unique three-dimensional chemical compounds on the cell membrane that interact with other chemicals and transmit the chemical signal to the nucleus of the cell. In the nucleus, the signal is interpreted by stimulating specific genes in the DNA template, which then become activated. When these PPAR-alpha receptors are activated by a diet rich in omega-3s, genes that help lower the inflammatory response of the body are activated.

OMEGA-3s REDUCE PRODUCTION OF INFLAMMATORY SUBSTANCES BY THE ARACHIDONIC ACID PATHWAY

Similar to the action of commonly used anti-inflammatory drugs such as Motrin and Naprosyn, omega-3 fats such as EPA and DHA, found in fish oils, affect important chemical steps in the arachidonic acid pathway. They lower the production of inflammatory compounds by shutting down the pathways that produce unhealthful prostaglandins, such as the LOX pathway.

CONCLUSIONS

1. Omega-3 fats have many beneficial effects in decreasing inflammation in our joints. They decrease the production of cartilage-degrading enzymes that are overproduced in osteoarthritis.
2. Omega-3 fats also turn off cartilage cell genes that code for inflammatory products.

3. Omega-3s inhibit the formation of toxic AGEs in the blood-stream by clearing sugar from the blood and storing it as glycogen for later use.
4. Omega-3s positively affect cartilage by helping maintain the proper three-dimensional structure of healthy cartilage.
5. Because of all these benefits, omega-3s are beneficial neu-traceuticals in the treatment of osteoarthritis.

FIGURE 9-1
BENEFICIAL EFFECTS OF OMEGA-3 FATS

1. They decrease clotting in the blood and make the blood thinner. This has benefits in decreasing the formation of blood clots, strokes, and heart attacks.

2. They decrease blood triglyceride level.

3. They decrease blood pressure.

4. They cause increase in the "good" blood lipid called HDL.

5. They fight inflammation by lowering the production of inflammatory substances in the body.

6. They improve mitochondrial function.

7. They decrease enlargement of fat cells around our waists.

8. They activate genes that help burn fat and lower the body's ability to form fat.

9. They decrease the storage of triglycerides in cells and thus help fight obesity.

10. When they are incorporated in the cell membrane in large numbers, they regulate the uptake of blood sugar and thus lower the amount of sugar in the bloodstream.

11. They turn off inflammatory genes and turn on the genes that fight inflammation in the body.

10
Unhealthy Diets Cause Hormonal Imbalance

FAT IS AN IMPORTANT HORMONE-PRODUCING ORGAN

The organs in our body that produce hormones are called **endocrine organs**. Recent research reveals that fat is an important endocrine organ. Hormones regulate our body's chemical balance, called **homeostasis**. In the case of obesity, the wrong hormones are produced by the fat around the waist. This inflammatory fat contributes to the increase of inflammation throughout the body.

Fat normally produces hormones called adipocytokines. Two important adipocytokines are leptin and adiponectin. These fat-derived cytokine hormones control fat and sugar metabolism in the body. Inflamed fat found in joints produces leptin and adiponectin, which play an important role in stimulating cartilage cells to produce cartilage-degrading enzymes and inflammatory compounds which lead to cartilage breakdown in osteoarthritis.[1]

THE ROLE OF LEPTIN IN INFLAMMATION AND OBESITY

Leptin is a hormone produced by fat cells. The levels of leptin and the inflammatory compounds IL-1 and TNF-alpha are increased in obese people.[2] Leptin interacts with cells to activate certain genes that have important regulatory effects on energy production, our body's inflammation state, and the development of insulin resistance.[3] A chemical compound called **SOCS-3**, which I will discuss in more detail in chapter 12, is important in blocking the signaling pathways of leptin.

Leptin acts through brain receptors in the **hypothalamus** to cause us to stop eating when we have consumed enough calories. The hypothalamus has a number of regulatory centers that control functions in the body such as breathing and hunger that are not under our conscious control. This important function of controlling hunger is regulated well when leptin functions normally, but when leptin is increased a state of leptin resistance develops and the hypothalamus does not respond appropriately to its signals. As a result, we continue to eat even when our body does not need the excess calories.

Leptin is critical to determining how fat is processed in the body[4] and how much inflammation is present in our bodies.[5] Genetic mutations have been found in the gene that codes for the leptin hormone that lead to the development of obesity, insulin resistance, and eventually type 2 diabetes. Leptin increases inflammation by increasing the production of inflammatory compounds by white blood cells.[6]

LEPTIN RESISTANCE

In people who are obese, leptin and insulin hormones are dysfunctional, making the body unable to properly hear the signals conveyed by these hormones. Obesity leads to increased circulating levels of leptin.[7] *A state of leptin resistance develops in obese people that, like insulin resistance, results in cells not responding to the messages of leptin.*[8] Studies have shown that people with metabolic syndrome have insulin resistance with elevated insulin blood levels. This elevated insulin leads to increased blood leptin and to leptin resistance.[9]

LEPTIN STIMULATES PRODUCTION OF INFLAMMATORY CYTOKINES AND NITRIC OXIDE

Leptin is overproduced by the "plump" fat cells in people with obesity;[10] it is also overproduced in arthritic cartilage cells. Increased leptin levels trigger an increase in the production of the inflammatory compound nitric oxide.[11] Nitric oxide is important in activating the genes in cartilage cells that produce inflammatory compounds and in also activating "suicide genes" that lead to cartilage cell death.[12]

Leptin also teams up with another cartilage villain, IL-1, to increase the production of nitric oxide. As discussed earlier, IL-1 is an important cytokine produced by osteoarthritic cartilage cells and inflamed fat found in the joints. Both IL-1 and nitric oxide activate genes in cartilage that increase the production of the cartilage-degrading MMPs. IL-1 stimulates another inflammatory substance, **oncostatin M**, to further increase MMP and another cartilage-degrading enzyme, **ADAMTS4**.[13] Thus a cycle of increasing cartilage destruction is generated.

LEPTIN LEVELS ARE ELEVATED IN OSTEOARTHRITIS AND OBESITY

Research has shown that cartilage cells contain the **leptin receptor** known as **Ob-R**.[14] In the absence of leptin resistance, leptin stimulates cartilage cells to increase their growth and the production of the three-dimensional collagen structure that gives cartilage its strength and resiliency.[15] When leptin is measured in the synovial fluid in cartilage taken from osteoarthritic patients, it is found to be elevated. *Obese patients with osteoarthritis have even higher leptin levels in their joints than nonobese osteoarthritic patients.*[16]

Research has found that the more obese a person with osteoarthritis is, the higher the level of leptin seen in their synovial joint fluid.[17] Leptin is not found in the joint fluid of normal, nonarthritic knees, and is only minimally produced in normal cartilage. Heavier people who are also osteoarthritic have increased leptin in both their joints and in the arthritic bone spurs that are often seen accompanying osteoarthritis.[18] Bone spurs are excess bone that develops in the joint adjacent to areas in which the cartilage cap that covers the bone has been worn down by osteoarthritis. *Osteoarthritis is more destructive in people with increased joint leptin levels.* On the other hand, normal leptin levels, as well as normally functioning leptin (i.e., without leptin resistance), have beneficial effects on cartilage, including increased production of IGF-1 and TGF-beta-1, which promote the proper building and maintenance of cartilage. An increase in leptin levels stimulates the production of inflammatory compounds. It is also known that women have higher circulating leptin levels than men do, and this may be a factor as to the reason obese women develop earlier onset and more aggressive damage in their knees from osteoarthritis than obese men do.

ADIPONECTIN PLAYS A ROLE IN OSTEOARTHRITIS

Adiponectin is a fat-derived hormone found in lower levels in obese than nonobese people.[19] Lowered adiponectin in obesity is associated with the development of insulin resistance and metabolic syndrome.[20] Researchers have shown that fat cells present in joints produce

FIGURE 10-1
DETRIMENTAL EFFECTS OF INCREASED LEPTIN
AND LEPTIN RESISTANCE ON JOINT CARTILAGE

✓ Obesity leads to increased leptin production and leptin resistance.

✓ Leptin increases production of inflammatory compounds (cytokines and NO).

✓ Leptin is increased in osteoarthritic joints.

✓ Obese osteoarthritic people have more leptin in their joints than nonobese osteoarthritic people.

✓ Leptin links the obesity epidemic to the development of osteoarthritis. (Leptin and IL-1 increase NO and cartilage breakdown.)

✓ Obese women have elevated leptin levels and a predisposition to early development of osteoarthritis.

adiponectin.[21] In osteoarthritic joints, adiponectin has been shown to have inflammatory effects by increasing the production of IL-6 and stimulating the production of cartilage-degrading MMPs.[22]

The gene that codes for adiponectin has been isolated, and has been shown to be very active in joints of osteoarthritic people. Adiponectin's role is currently not completely clear and is being explored in attempts to determine how it is involved in cartilage breakdown.

THE PROPER FUNCTIONING OF INSULIN FIGHTS INFLAMMATION IN THE BODY

Insulin, when functioning normally and in its proper blood levels, has beneficial anti-inflammatory and antioxidant properties. Properly functioning insulin suppresses the important inflammatory message

FIGURE 10-2
INFLAMMATORY CYTOKINES PRODUCED IN KNEE FAT

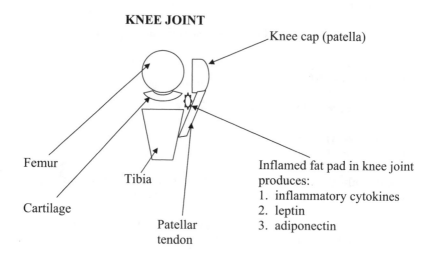

relay station NFkB, which turns on harmful genes in cartilage cells. Insulin also acts to decrease the formation of oxygen free radicals, which harm cartilage, and also decreases the production of inflammatory compounds IL-6 and TNF-alpha.[23]

INSULIN RESISTANCE SKYROCKETS THE PRODUCTION OF FREE RADICALS

Insulin resistance increases inflammation in our bodies, leading to the development of metabolic syndrome.[24] It also increases the production of oxygen free radicals, leading to increased oxidative stress.[25] Oxygen free radicals attack the cell membrane and cause its components to become rancid, or oxidized. This results in leakage of the membrane and toxin accumulation in cells. Free radicals also activate NFkB, triggering inflammation. Excess blood sugar itself directly stimulates NFkB and turns on inflammatory genes in cells. It also stimulates another important cell enzyme, **NADPH oxidase**, which forms more free radicals.

INCREASED INFLAMMATION AND INSULIN RESISTANCE LEAD TO HORMONAL IMBALANCES

People with increased levels of insulin and sugar in their blood have more inflammation and also have higher production of **cortisol**. Cortisol is the hormone produced by the **adrenal glands**, which sit on top of the kidneys, and is involved in the "fight-or-flight" response. It is a stress hormone that is increased in situations of physical or emotional stress. Chronic elevation of stress is harmful to the body. In a state of constant stress and inflammation, the excess production of cortisol leads to muscle breakdown and increased blood sugar levels. Excess cortisol also increases insulin levels, which leads to a vicious cycle of increase in the fat around the waist. Other harmful effects include an increase in production of arachidonic acid and a decrease in testosterone. If stress is not controlled, a condition referred to as *adrenal burnout* eventually develops, resulting in the inability of the adrenal gland to produce its hormones at appropriate levels.

THE ROLE OF SNPS AND GENETIC INDIVIDUALITY

New research in genetics has identified small changes in the genes— SNPs—of important inflammatory compounds that predispose individuals with a particular SNP to increased inflammation and damage. This highlights the genetic individuality among different people and their different responses to the environment and what they eat.

FIGURE 10-3
DETRIMENTAL EFFECTS OF INSULIN RESISTANCE

1. Increased inflammation in the body

2. Hormonal imbalances

3. Cartilage breakdown in joints

4. Development of obesity

5. Leptin resistance

6. Increased formation of damaging free radicals in our joints

7. Development of metabolic syndrome

Genetic studies have shown that the IL-6 gene contains an SNP that predisposes people possessing it to a much higher incidence of insulin resistance. The fat-produced adiponectin hormone is coded by a gene that has an SNP known as the 276 G-T SNP. Carriers of this particular SNP have a higher propensity to developing oxidative stress in their bodies. Leptin, another fat-produced hormone, is coded for by the Ob gene. Research has shown that mutations in the gene that codes for leptin cause obesity and high blood pressure in both humans and animals.

OBESITY PREDISPOSES WOMEN TO INCREASED LEPTIN LEVELS AND TO OSTEOARTHRITIS

New scientific evidence—as well as my personal experience of patients being seen for osteoarthritis—suggests that osteoarthritis is more common in women than men.[26] Studies have also shown that obese women have a higher incidence than obese men of knee osteoarthritis development and progression at a younger age. Leptin has been shown by researchers to be actively involved in osteoarthritic joint damage,[27] and women have higher leptin levels than men.[28]

There seems to be a correlation of obese women, increased leptin levels, and the propensity to develop earlier onset osteoarthritis. The Framingham study (a large study initiated in 1948 by the National Institutes of Health to study the causes of heart disease and stroke has followed large groups of patients [including families with grandparents, parents, and children] over time to determine how risk factors such as obesity, hypertension, smoking, and genetics play a role in the development of heart disease) showed that in overweight females, losing only eleven pounds decreased the risk of symptomatic knee osteoarthritis by 50 percent.[29] Furthermore, hand osteoarthritis, which involves non-weight-bearing joints, positively correlates with obesity.[30] Hand joints are not subjected to the same mechanical stresses as knees and hips, so their association with obesity is the result of chemical and hormonal causes as opposed to excessive weight "mechanically" causing the breakdown of joints. These findings support the theory that osteoarthritis is a disorder contributed to by metabolic dysfunction in the body.

ESTROGEN RECEPTORS, MENOPAUSE, AND OSTEOARTHRITIS

The female hormone estrogen is an important regulator of cartilage cells, and women have a higher incidence of osteoarthritis compared to men. Cartilage cells have estrogen receptors on their surfaces, and female cartilage cells, more than male cartilage cells, when stimulated by estrogen, increase the production of cartilage repair enzymes and components of the cartilage framework. Estrogen has other beneficial effects in the body by stimulating the burning of fats, activating the anti-inflammatory message relay station **PPAR-delta**, and preventing the formation of fat. Menopause results in decreased levels of estrogen, which can be detrimental to joint cartilage. Women with hormonal imbalances caused by obesity and increased blood sugar levels are especially at risk for developing osteoarthritis.[31] Results from the Framingham study have shown that women with higher **bone mineral density (BMD)**, and thus stronger bones, have a decreased risk of progression of their osteoarthritis.[32] *Menopause, with its relative estrogen deficiency and increased fat formation, results in weakening of the bones of women and also increased risk of developing osteoarthritis and other metabolic diseases.* It is important to note that increased fat decreases the strength of bone. While it is true that a higher body mass is correlated with stronger bones, when the fat percentage of total body mass is looked at it correlates with weakening of bones. Thus being overweight is both detrimental to both bone and cartilage.

CONCLUSIONS

1. The hormonal and metabolic status of our bodies has an important effect on the development of osteoarthritis.
2. The maintenance of optimum insulin levels in the bloodstream and optimum insulin functioning are important in combating cartilage destruction in osteoarthritis. Poor nutrition generates a cycle of hormonal imbalance that negatively affects the whole body.
3. Middle-aged women who are also obese have a high risk of developing progressive knee osteoarthritis.
4. Obese women have increased leptin levels, decreased estrogen, and metabolically active obese fat cells, all of which interact to increase the inflammation in their bodies and lead to osteoarthritic cartilage breakdown.
5. Estrogen is an important regulator of cartilage cells, and its decrease in menopause predisposes to osteoarthritis.
6. Osteoarthritis changes the chemical activity of cartilage cells by turning on genes that code for inflammatory compounds,

and increases production of cartilage-degrading MMPs.

7. Obesity is related to osteoarthritis development through high leptin levels and leptin resistance.

8. Leptin resistance, combined with increased leptin levels in the blood and in the joints, is associated with greater cartilage destruction in osteoarthritic joints.

9. Obese people with insulin resistance and metabolic syndrome also have leptin resistance.

10. The detrimental hormonal effects of leptin resistance occur in obesity, pre-diabetes, and osteoarthritis. They provide a common link connecting the obesity epidemic with pre-diabetes and osteoarthritis.

11. Leptin is a key regulator of cartilage cell function and activity.

12. Leptin resistance and increased leptin production are important factors in the progression of osteoarthritis.

13. Leptin activates white blood cells to produce inflammatory products, stimulates the production of nitric oxide, increases inflammatory cytokine production by cartilage cells, and acts to activate the immune system. These actions increase cartilage destruction in osteoarthritis.

14. Leptin is produced excessively in people with metabolic syndrome and obesity.

15. Leptin forms an important bridge linking obesity, metabolic syndrome, poor nutrition, and the development of osteoarthritis.

16. SNPs in the Ob gene coding for leptin, adiponectin, and IL-6 predispose certain people to increased oxidative stress, insulin resistance, and the development of osteoarthritis.

17. Inflammatory diets high in sugar and saturated and trans fats lead to insulin and leptin resistance. These events trigger cartilage destruction in the joints of susceptible people by interfering with the normal cartilage repair and maintenance system.

11

Sweet Toxins That Destroy Our Joints: How AGEs Lead to Osteoarthritis

RAGE AND OSTEOARTHRITIS

O steoarthritic cartilage cells are not normal in appearance. They are stimulated to become bigger in size. They also become more chemically active and start producing chemicals and enzymes that break down cartilage.[1]

Recent research has shown that an important mechanism by which normal cartilage cells become "plump" is by activation of a special receptor on their cell surface known as RAGE.[2] The AGE-RAGE "lock-in-key" complex initiates a whole series of harmful reactions in our joints that lead to decreased production of collagen (the building block protein of cartilage) and disruption of the normal three-dimensional structure of cartilage.[3] As described earlier, this is seen in the weak, fragile, yellowish cartilage present in osteoarthritis. Normal, healthy cartilage, on the other hand, has a pristine white colored appearance.

FIGURE 11-1
CAUSES OF ENLARGED CARTILAGE CELLS
IN OSTEOARTHRITIS

1.   Excess inflammation in the body

2.   The aging process

3.   Sugar-coated proteins, produced as a result of chronically elevated blood sugar levels and high incidence of metabolic syndrome

SUGAR-COATED PROTEINS AND OSTEOARTHRITIS

The modern American diet, high in sugar and unhealthy refined carbohydrates (such as white bread and pasta), results in chronically elevated blood sugar levels. People with such high blood sugar levels are in a state of pre-diabetes, and damaging sugar-coated AGEs accumulate in their organs. *These AGEs are very resistant to breakdown by the body and tend to accumulate and get deposited in our joints.*

As AGEs accumulate in joints, they damage the cartilage and cause it to deteriorate. Researchers have found elevated AGE levels in the blood and joint fluid of osteoarthritic patients.[4] An unhealthy diet also causes acidosis (low pH) and low oxygen content in our organs. The body does not function well with a low pH and under low oxygen conditions. As a result, oxidative stress increases, which increases the number of oxygen free radicals that damage cells and organs. In a vicious cycle, these conditions further increase the formation of AGEs. A healthy diet high in omega-3 fats and antioxidants decreases the amount of AGEs in the blood and is beneficial for joint health.

The AGE-RAGE interaction directly turns on genes in cartilage cells, which results in increased inflammation, increased cellular acidity, and increased cell damage.[5] Furthermore, "suicide genes" are turned on, releasing toxic chemicals that kill the cartilage cell from the inside out.[6] When a cartilage cell dies, it stops manufacturing and replenishing the collagen framework that makes up the cartilage cushion in our joints. The cartilage cushion then begins to crumble and disintegrate, resulting in osteoarthritis.

GLYCATED COLLAGEN RESULTS IN WEAKER JOINTS

As we have already seen, collagen is a three-dimensional protein that forms the backbone of cartilage. Within this cartilage backbone are located the cartilage cells, which are laced across the collagen surface in a pattern similar to stars on the canvas of an evening sky.

The cartilage matrix is an organ that lacks blood vessels, lymph drainage, and nerve endings. The lymphatic system is the pipe drainage and filtering system of the body; because it is not present in cartilage, toxins, rust-forming compounds, and acidic wastes that become built up in the body due to poor nutrition, aging, and environmental toxins are able to accumulate there. In osteoarthritis, sugar-coated AGEs circulating in the blood are deposited in the joint and bind to collagen in the cartilage. The resulting **glycated collagen** has been shown in studies to be weaker, stiffer, and less resilient to stresses than collagen in normal cartilage,[7] leading to its breakdown and the development of osteoarthritis.

Stiff, sugar-coated cartilage has increased levels of cartilage-breakdown enzymes.[8] It also stimulates the secretion of inflammatory substances, the cytokines, which further damage the cartilage. A cycle is thus created of increased cartilage breakdown, resulting in pain, swelling, and deformity of the joint. These are some of the mechanisms by which poor nutrition leads to cartilage breakdown and osteoarthritis.[9]

OXIDATIVE STRESS STIMULATES RAGE RECEPTOR ACTIVATION IN CARTILAGE CELLS

Increased oxidative stress stimulates the RAGE receptor gene to increase the production of the RAGE receptor and amplify the inflammation.[10] It also leads to production of more **hydrogen peroxide (H_2O_2)**. Hydrogen peroxide is a caustic chemical that damages cartilage cells. Fats in the blood, when exposed to increased sugar concentrations, become sugar coated and oxidized. This oxidation of fats makes them more toxic and more inflammatory.[11] Sugar-coated fats also interact with RAGE receptors and further propagate inflammation.

COOKING AT HIGH TEMPERATURES CAUSES THE FORMATION OF AGEs

One interesting finding is that food cooked at high temperatures leads to increased AGE formation.[12] Higher cooking temperatures have also been found to increase inflammation. Research has shown that broiling meat at 437°F (225°C) and frying at 350°F (177°C) results in the highest levels of AGEs.[13] Boiling in high heat also increases the "sugar-coating" and oxidation of common foods, thus making them more inflammatory.

Eating foods with large amounts of sugars (**high-glycemic-load diets**) leads to high AGE production, and this, along with cooking foods at high temperatures, is unhealthy and accelerates the aging process.[14]

AGEs CAUSE CARTILAGE DESTRUCTION

Recent research has shown that when AGEs build up in the blood, the risk of developing osteoarthritis is increased. Animals with osteoarthritis in their joints responded to increased amounts of AGEs by developing a more aggressive form of osteoarthritis.[15] Other studies have shown that when cartilage cells are exposed to AGEs, they increase their number of RAGE receptors. This in turn leads to these cells producing the cartilage breakdown enzymes called MMPs.[16]

AGEs have another detrimental effect on the body: they decrease the normal function of the detoxifying enzymes catalase, glutathione peroxidase, and superoxide dismutase. These are the engines that drive the toxic cleanup in our cells and organs. When these enzymes do not work properly, the environment inside the cells becomes polluted with acidic wastes and oxygen free radicals. When they malfunction in cartilage as a result of the overaccumulation of AGEs, the toxic buildup in the joint becomes excessive and causes cartilage damage.

FIGURE 11-2
RAGE AND CARTILAGE DESTRUCTION

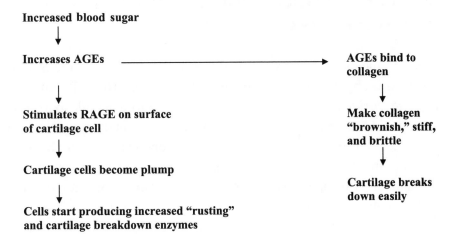

Increased blood sugar
↓
Increases AGEs ⟶ AGEs bind to collagen
↓ ↓
Stimulates RAGE on surface of cartilage cell / Make collagen "brownish," stiff, and brittle
↓ ↓
Cartilage cells become plump / Cartilage breaks down easily
↓
Cells start producing increased "rusting" and cartilage breakdown enzymes

RAGE ACTIVATES THE INFLAMMATION-PRODUCING PATHWAYS

RAGE receptors[17] have the ability to bind a number of compounds from their surrounding environment. When sugar-coated AGEs activate these receptors, inflammation is increased.[18] Hydrogen peroxide and oxygen free radicals, which cause oxidative stress, are stimulated by RAGE. The increased oxidative stress environment caused by RAGE also activates "suicide genes," as well causing the activation of the important signal relay intermediate NFkB.[19]

RAGE activation by AGEs also results in increased production of the inflammatory arachidonic acid, which is the precursor of the inflammatory prostaglandins.[20] Prostaglandins are responsible for the swelling, pain, and redness that occur when our joints are inflamed. Minimizing the production of arachidonic acid is important in controlling unwanted inflammation in the body. **N-acetylcysteine (NAC)** is an important, potent antioxidant that has the ability to reduce arachidonic acid production and can be taken as a supplement.[21]

THE RAGE RECEPTOR GENE DIFFERS AMONG PEOPLE, DETERMINING THE DAMAGE CAUSED BY RAGE

Recent studies have shown that the gene that codes for the RAGE receptor is slightly different from person to person. This difference, or *genetic variability*, is in the form of a single nucleotide polymorphism.[22] As discussed previously, an SNP is a small change in the sequence that forms the gene. People with one particular SNP variation are more prone than other people to experiencing an aggressive inflammatory response when exposed to high-sugar-content foods and sugar-coated proteins.

A recently discovered SNP in the RAGE gene is called **G82S**.

People with this G82S SNP produce a RAGE receptor that is more aggressive in triggering cartilage destruction and inflammation in the joints.[23] This SNP triggers the production of increased levels of cartilage-degrading MMPs, and when people who have it consume an unhealthy, high-sugar diet, they are more prone to developing cartilage damage.

RAGE AFFECTS BONE

RAGE has an important function in regulating normal bone turnover. When RAGE is activated excessively by AGEs, it overstimulates the osteoclasts that break down bone.[24] This causes the bone changes seen in osteoarthritis, including weakened and dysfunctional bone.

CONCLUSIONS

1. RAGE activation by AGEs causes cartilage cells to change appearance, becoming plumper and more active. This change results in the activation of chemical processes in cartilage that lead to the excessive production of inflammatory substances, oxygen free radicals, and cartilage-breakdown enzymes. Cartilage cell enlargement is analogous to fat cell enlargement seen in obesity, pre-diabetes, and metabolic syndrome. Increased inflammation, acidity, and "rusting" all occur, conspiring to cause cartilage damage in osteoarthritis.
2. Osteoarthritic cartilage has increased levels of both RAGE receptors and MMPs.
3. Increased oxidative stress leads to cartilage damage. AGEs stimulate the RAGE receptor, leading to increased oxidative stress.
4. Chronically elevated blood sugar, as seen in people with pre-diabetes and metabolic syndrome, activates the RAGE receptors.

5. Collagen, the building block of cartilage, combines with AGEs and other acidic wastes. This weakens the collagen and causes it to collapse under normal, everyday stresses. This leads to cartilage destruction in our joints.

6. DNA can undergo sugar coating as a result of chronically excessive blood sugar levels. This causes the DNA to malfunction and genes are not appropriately activated and deactivated.

7. Chronically elevated systemic inflammation directly affects our genes. Inflammation turns on genes that cause cartilage cells to become "plump" and overproduce cartilage-degrading chemicals and enzymes.

8. Increased sugar consumption in our diet leads to activation of the NFkB signal intermediate relay station, causing increased production of free radicals and rust. These toxins trigger further inflammatory genes to be turned on and produce MMPs. This is a powerful example of how our diet affects our genes and leads to cartilage destruction in osteoarthritis.

9. Improving our diet with foods low in sugar and high in antioxidants and omega-3 fats decreases AGE production and helps keep our cartilage healthy.

10. A high-sugar diet directly affects the size and shape of cartilage cells through the formation of AGEs and their interaction with the RAGE receptors. This is a very powerful concept that links diet, its affects on altering the body's metabolism, and the development of osteoarthritis.

12

Why It Is Not a Good Idea to Treat Osteoarthritis with Drugs

WHAT IS THE PROBLEM WITH DRUGS?

There are many complex biochemical reactions involved in maintaining normal cartilage health in our joints. From my professional experience with the numerous drugs used in the treatment of osteoarthritis, it is unlikely that any drug that uses a "single-bullet" approach to attacking a particular chemical reaction in cartilage cells will lead to a cure for arthritis. One of the problems with using drugs to treat osteoarthritis is that they target complex pathways in the body that, when blocked in different organ systems by the drug, are likely to lead to side effects. Furthermore, they are unable to affect the underlying causes of osteoarthritis. The drugs currently used to treat osteoarthritis—nonsteroidal anti-inflammatories, steroid injections, and painkillers—do nothing to alter the course of the disease or provide a cure. They are effective in treating pain symptoms, but at a heavy price! Even though drugs cannot cure arthritis, because they block chemical reactions across many different organs in the body, they can have detrimental effects in organs other than the "target organ" they are intended to affect. These unwanted side effects are the reason drug interactions are a leading cause of death and toxicity in this country.

THE POPULAR NONSTEROIDAL DRUGS AND THEIR SIDE EFFECTS

An example of unwanted drug consequences is found in the case of the popular nonsteroidal anti-inflammatories, the COX-2 inhibitors. These include Vioxx and Bextra, which were recently pulled off the market. Vioxx and Bextra were beneficial in the treatment of pain and inflammation in arthritis by blocking the formation of inflammatory prostaglandins in the arachidonic acid pathway. While these drugs were never shown to be able to cure or reverse osteoarthritis, they did have side effects in other organs. The enzyme they block, COX-2, is found in many other organ systems in the body, and while blocking it helped arthritic pain, it had detrimental effects on the heart. The removal of these once very popular arthritic drugs from the market is more evidence of the need for a fresh approach when attacking complex degenerative diseases such as osteoarthritis. We must develop a more holistic approach in treating this disease by employing nutritional and nutraceutical strategies that do not have the dangerous side effects of nonsteroidal drugs.

WHY ARE ANTI-INFLAMMATORY DRUGS DANGEROUS TO CARTILAGE IN OUR JOINTS?

The interest in using nutritional methods to combat osteoarthritis is borne out of physicians' and patients' experiences with the widely used nonsteroidal anti-inflammatory drugs. Nonsteroidals currently play a major role in the treatment of osteoarthritis. They act by blocking the arachidonic acid pathway and thus decreasing the synthesis of inflammatory prostaglandins. This approach is associated with unwanted side effects because prostaglandins are involved in complex pathways that have positive as well as negative effects on joint cartilage and other organs. While the short-term use of these drugs is appropriate and has beneficial effects in decreasing the pain and inflammation associated with osteoarthritis, they have never been proven in scientific research studies to have any **disease-modifying benefits**.

Aspirin is widely used for pain relief in osteoarthritic patients. Aspirin inhibits the enzymes involved in the early stages of cartilage manufacturing. This is a drawback to aspirin use. Several nonsteroidal anti-inflammatories also suppress the synthesis of the proteoglycans that make up the cartilage backbone. The depletion of these important cartilage subunits is a major reason nonsteroidals can be toxic to the already damaged joint cartilage found in patients with osteoarthritis.[1] In one scientific study, researchers studied thirteen different nonsteroidal drugs available in the market for use with osteoarthritis and compared their effects on cartilage cells. Arthritic cartilage is more prone than normal cartilage to damage from nonsteroidals because diseased cartilage cells do not function well and accumulate the drug, amplifying side effects. Please refer back to the discussion in chapter 1.

NONSTEROIDAL ANTI-INFLAMMATORY DRUGS ARE RESPONSIBLE FOR SIGNIFICANT COMPLICATIONS

Each year, more than 100,000 people are admitted to hospitals as a result of gastrointestinal complications brought on by nonsteroidal anti-inflammatory use. Of those, 15 percent—mostly elderly—die from their gastrointestinal problems. That is a total of about 16,500 deaths per year in the United States caused by complications from properly prescribed and properly taken nonsteroidal anti-inflammatories. In patients greater than sixty-five years of age, researchers have shown that up to 30 percent of hospital admissions and deaths from nonsteroidal drug complications are the result of stomach ulcers.[2] This is because the drugs block the COX-1 enzyme, which is present in stomach cells as well as in cartilage cells in joints. Blocking this enzyme in the stomach is bad, as it results in the development of ulcers.

In the remainder of this chapter I will discuss the risks associated with newer classes of drugs that are currently either being developed or are already in use. This discussion will make clear that nutritional and nutraceutical treatment of osteoarthritis is a much safer approach. Drugs have a proper place in the treatment of advanced osteoarthritis when they are used for short periods of time, but they should not be the first and last line of attack, as is currently the standard of practice.

PPAR ACTIVATORS AND NFKB INHIBITORS

Pharmaceutical companies are developing drugs to manipulate the NFkB and PPAR pathways described earlier in this book.[3] NFkB is the inflammatory compound that is the signal intermediate for many of the inflammatory and cartilage-breakdown chemicals generated in osteoarthritis. PPAR receptors are beneficial receptors that block the action of NFkB and thus generate anti-inflammatory signals sent to the cell's DNA.

Recent efforts to develop PPAR activators, which are laboratory-manufactured drugs intended to stimulate the PPAR receptor, have resulted in the production of drugs that have been shown to produce significant liver damage. Rather than using these new drugs, which have been found to be toxic, the approach I am recommending is to activate the PPAR receptors with proper nutrition and the use of safe nutraceuticals. The omega-3 fats EPA and DHA, two active ingredients in fish oils, are potent PPAR receptor activators. They do not have the side effects of drugs, and they can be purchased over the counter. There are also biologically active plant compounds in such vegetables as broccoli and kale that have been shown to stimulate PPAR-gamma receptors. They have beneficial effects on lowering blood sugar and blood lipid levels without the side effects of drugs. Plant nutritional substances can be taken in concentrated supplement form and are found in most health food stores. It is wise to use well-known brands from large, reputable manufacturers.

Steroids, which were developed in the 1950s, act in part by blocking the damaging action of NFkB and preventing cells from manufacturing inflammatory and toxic compounds that lead to oxidative stress. Unfortunately, steroids also have dangerous side effects. While they are effective in decreasing the pain and inflammation of osteoarthritis, they do not alter the course of the disease. Given in large doses and for prolonged periods of time, steroids accelerate the progression of arthritis by promoting cartilage deterioration.

The PPAR and NFkB systems in the body are very complex, and their receptors behave differently in different organs and under different chemical conditions. This is why it is dangerous to try to influence these systems with the use of laboratory-manufactured drugs, which have blanket effect on all receptors in all organs in the body. *Because of their potency and nonselectivity, drugs lead to side effects in unintended organs.*

MMP INHIBITORS

Matrix metalloproteinases are important cartilage-degrading enzymes that are overproduced and are overactive in osteoarthritis, causing much of the cartilage destruction seen in this disease. The pharmaceutical industry is attempting to find laboratory-manufactured drugs to block the production of these cartilage-degrading enzymes.[4] The danger in this approach lies in the fact that MMPs are needed, in optimal levels, for the normal "housekeeping" functions, not just in cartilage but in connective tissues in other organs in the body. The assembly and remodeling of the three-dimensional cartilage matrix by cartilage cells are aided by the proper functioning of a very important MMP, MMP-13. Researchers have shown that mice that are deficient in MMP-13 exhibit defective bone development, abnormal skeleton growth, and deformities.[5] Other researchers have shown that when the MMP-13 gene was experimentally removed from the DNA of mice, they developed deadly clots in their blood vessels similar to those seen in people having heart attacks. These MMP-13-deficient mice had thinner and less well-organized collagen on the walls and in the plaque of their vessels.[6] Vessels can accumulate sludge called plaque, which is the culprit in blocking blood flow, leading to strokes and heart attacks. One interesting finding was that the plaque in the vessel walls of these mice was itself weak as a result of the defective collagen caused by their gene defect. These plaques made of weak collagen break off more easily. This is why these mice had higher numbers of deadly heart attacks and other clotting events.

The above studies highlight the fact that an across-the-board drug blockade of these enzymes is likely to disrupt the normal function and maintenance of bone and blood vessels, leading to unwanted side effects. Used in humans, a drug that blocks MMP-13 production will have similar effects to those seen in the mice described above.

The indiscriminate action of drugs, through their blanket effect on a particular enzyme system across many different organs in the body, is often accompanied by dangerous side effects.

MMP INHIBITOR DRUGS ARE TOXIC

All the MMP inhibitor drugs tested thus far in clinical trials have been found to promote toxicity in major organ systems. The antibiotic doxycycline is the only MMP inhibitor that has been used without short-term toxicity.[7] The long-term effects of doxycycline are unknown, as antibiotics have toxic effects on the gastrointestinal tract by killing off beneficial bacteria. Attempts are being made to modify doxycycline and make it more "stomach friendly" while still preserving its ability to block MMPs.

TNF-ALPHA- AND IL-1-BLOCKING AGENTS

TNF-alpha and IL-1 are the inflammatory and toxic cytokines that play an important role in the destruction of cartilage in osteoarthritis. TNF-alpha- and IL-1-blocking drugs are currently being used to treat rheumatoid arthritis. Recent follow-up studies done on these drugs have been released, showing that rheumatoid arthritis patients treated with these drugs have increased susceptibility to developing opportunistic lung infections[8] and cancer.[9] This is a result of the adverse effects these drugs have on the immune system. In 2006, researchers reported that randomized, controlled clinical trials involving the TNF-alpha inhibitors Remicade and Humira showed a dose-related increased risk of cancer development.[10] Another research group reported increased risk of developing lymphoma, which is cancer of the blood, with the use of TNF-alpha-blocking drugs.[11] We must not negate the benefits of these drugs in treating severe cases of rheumatoid arthritis. What I am proposing is using safer nutraceutical approaches whenever possible.

RANKL INHIBITORS

RANKL is an important enzyme system found in bone that is responsible for the proper maintenance of bone mass and of remodeling.[12] Activation of RANKL receptors activates bone cells called osteoclasts, which break down bone. Its action is opposed by **osteoprote-**

gerin (OPG), which blocks osteoclasts. Other bone cells, called osteoblasts, are responsible for building new bone. In order for the body to maintain proper bone density, it is necessary to keep a finely tuned balance of osteoblast and osteoclast action, which is controlled by the OPG/RANKL chemical enzyme system.

Researchers have found that both immune cells and bone cells contain RANKL. The activation of RANKL by white blood cells in arthritis is thought to contribute to the bone loss observed in patients with arthritis. Drug companies are trying to develop drugs that block RANKL in order to prevent cartilage breakdown in the treatment of osteoporosis. Because TNF and RANKL are involved in the normal bone remodeling, using drugs to block them in order to treat osteoarthritis can be expected to have detrimental effects on bone. This may result in creating brittle, hardened bones that are prone to breaking. In the effort to control cartilage damage, the result may lead to the development of bone diseases.

DRUGS THAT TARGET iNOS AND NADPH OXIDASE

Researchers are attempting to develop drugs that target iNOS, the enzyme involved in the formation of nitric oxide, an inflammatory compound involved in cartilage damage.[13] Nitric oxide is a powerful oxidant that triggers inflammation and oxidative stress in joint cartilage. Nitric oxide has different effects in different organs in the body. It is beneficial in blood vessels, but detrimental in joint cartilage. Therefore, using a drug to block it may help cartilage while risking damage to blood vessels.

Oxidative stress is produced by oxygen free radicals generated by mitochondria in the normal process of turning food into energy. Oxygen free radicals in turn activate NFkB, which turns on inflammatory genes. Drugs are being developed to target the **mitochondrial electron transport chain**, which produces energy, and the important enzyme NADPH oxidase. The potential risk is that by "knocking out" the important maintenance and energy-producing systems with an indiscriminate, across-the-board drug blockade is likely to cause serious side effects and unintended collateral damage. All drugs have side effects. Some drugs never make it past animal or human studies because of their serious side effects.

ADAMTS INHIBITORS

Pharmaceutical companies are also targeting the **ADAMTS** enzyme system, attempting to design drugs that inhibit its normal functioning.[14] The ADAMTS enzyme system is important for normal maintenance functions in the body. It has differing functions depending on the local environment of the organ it is found in, such as local acidity (pH), biochemical environment, and its interaction with other active compounds. ADAMTS in cartilage has different function than in the cardiovascular system. While it may be beneficial to block ADAMTS in cartilage to prevent further breakdown, blocking it in the cardiovascular system is an unintended consequence of the drug. The use of drugs, such as ADAMTS inhibitors, in the treatment of osteoarthritis do not show great potential, because they are likely to have many undesirable side effects.

A drug that knocks out an enzyme system such as ADAMTS in a blanket fashion and indiscriminately across many different organs has great potential to produce unwanted side effects. These enzyme systems are important to many functions in the body. An across-the-board inhibition by a drug is likely to cause collateral damage similar to that seen with the COX-2 inhibitors Vioxx and Bextra. Many of these drugs are only in testing phase and their full side effects are not known yet.

RAGE BLOCKADE DRUGS

Drug company researchers are attempting to synthesize compounds that will bind to and block RAGE receptors.[15] This has the potential for serious and unforeseen side effects because RAGE receptors are a broad class of receptors that normally bind a large number of different compounds. If all the RAGE receptors in the body were blocked by a drug, the beneficial interactions between RAGE and its binding compounds would be negatively affected. A number of drugs have undergone early preliminary testing as inhibitors of advanced glycation endproduct formation,[16] including the drug ALT-711, which is active in breaking down protein cross-linking, and the drugs pyridoxamine and aminoguanidine. Studies with these are too preliminary and results are not available yet.

BIPHOSPHONATES AND OSTEOARTHRITIS

Biphosphonates are drugs that prevent the breakdown of bone and are normally used to treat osteoporosis. Researchers have used them in osteoarthritis in an effort to reverse some of the bone destruction seen with this disease. Biphosphonates block the increased bone turnover and excessive remodeling seen in the active stages of osteoarthritis. Early research studies looking at biphosphonates as a potential treatment for osteoarthritis have had mixed results. These drugs carry a number of side effects, including the recently publicized damage from bone cell death in the jaws of people taking the drug[17] as well as ulcers and damage to the esophagus and stomach.

MANIPULATING LEPTIN WITH DRUGS TO TREAT OSTEOARTHRITIS

Leptin resistance is a condition that affects many Americans who are afflicted with metabolic syndrome and obesity. A chemical compound called SOCS-3 is important in blocking the signaling pathways of leptin. Pharmaceutical companies are developing drugs to target SOCS-3 in order to manipulate leptin in the body. We have learned that leptin is overproduced in those who are obese and in osteoarthritic cartilage by fat cells in the joint, playing an important role in promoting the destruction of cartilage in osteoarthritis. But drugs targeting SOCS-3 will likely result in collateral damage. Because drugs are known to cause side effects, they should be used only as a last resort for treatment.

In this chapter, I have argued that drugs should not be the first line of attack on osteoarthritis, because they will probably only treat symptoms while having significant negative side effects. According to current experience, osteoarthritic drugs will have no effect on altering the course of the disease. The nutritional manipulation of leptin outlined in this book is a much safer approach to take. Even simple caloric restriction has very powerful effects, with studies in animals showing that calorically restricted animals live up to 30 to 40 percent longer than ones that are overfed. Caloric restriction in rheumatoid arthritis patients was found to improve the inflammatory profile by decreasing leptin, C-reactive protein, and the activation of white blood cells. The nutritional treatment of leptin resistance can reverse this metabolic abnormality without the side effects which are inherent in using drugs.

CONCLUSIONS

1. The biochemical pathways involved in causing metabolic dysfunction, inflammation, and oxidative stress are interconnected in the body.

2. Using drugs to target these pathways, which blocks them non-selectively and across the board in many different organ systems, is likely to cause serious side effects.

3. Drugs will not provide a "magic-bullet" cure for osteoarthritis.

4. The indiscriminate action of drugs, through their blanket effect on a particular enzyme system across many different organs in the body, is often accompanied by dangerous side effects.

5. This chapter highlights the potential detrimental effects of using drugs to target enzyme systems in the complex biochemical pathways of metabolic and degenerative joint disease. The use of nutraceuticals and nutritional treatments has been shown by research to be a powerful and effective way of addressing metabolic dysfunction. Future research needs to focus on better defining and validating the use of these new and exciting treatments.

6. The indiscriminate action of drugs in blocking a particular enzyme in many different organs other than the intended organ is a major drawback of drugs and also the reason they are plagued with side effects.

7. Natural substances such as nutraceuticals decrease NFkB but not as powerfully as drugs do. This more moderate inhibition of NFkB by nutraceuticals causes them to have less side effects compared to drugs. Active nutraceuticals that have been shown to block NFkB include alpha lipoic acid, vitamin E, curcumin, green tea bioflavonoids, and resveratrol in red wine. The omega-3 fats EPA and DHA found in fish oils are potent PPAR receptor activators that are much safer than drugs.

8. Overall, the current research on the use of MMP inhibitors in joint cartilage diseases has not been promising. The toxicity of these drugs highlight the potentially grave side effects of using drugs to block MMPs in the treatment of osteoarthritis.

9. The nutritional approaches to limiting the formation of AGEs and blocking RAGE receptors outlined in this book are much safer.

Part 3

NUTRIENTS BENEFICIAL TO OUR JOINTS

13

New Genetic Research Is Unraveling the Mysteries of Osteoarthritis

THE EFFECTS OF NUTRITION ON OUR GENES

Nutrition is an important environmental factor that affects our genes by mechanisms currently being unraveled by scientists.[1] Our nutrition is able to change the makeup of our DNA in a process called **epigenetic modification**.[2] In epigenetic modification, chemical changes (such as methylation) occur in segments of DNA that influence the adjacent genes to be either turned off or turned on. Therefore, this is equivalent to changing our genetic makeup. This powerful concept is central to the mechanisms by which our nutrition can change our DNA. Some genes are activated and others are deactivated by chemical changes in their sequence triggered by our diet. One such chemical change that occurs is called **methylation**. The addition of simple compounds composed of carbon and **hydrogen**, called methyl groups, to our DNA adjacent certain genes can lead to those genes being either activated or not. Increased inflammation and advanced glycation end-products generated by poor diets change the expression of genes by chemically modifying them.[3] This very powerful concept explains how the environment can shape our genetic makeup.[4] This genetic modification of our DNA caused by nutritional choices we make has an effect on our joint cartilage. New research is showing that poor nutrition and environmental toxins cause changes in our DNA that are passed on to our children.[5]

The inflammatory compounds such as IL-1 and TNF-alpha, which we discussed previously, are able to regulate the function of the gene in cartilage cells that codes for the cartilage-degrading MMPs.[6] In obesity the fat cells in the waist become enlarged and produce these inflammatory compounds. These in turn increase the production of MMPs by cartilage cells, leading to the breakdown of cartilage in osteoarthritis. The gene stimulation occurs by the intermediate signal relay station compounds such as NFkB and MAPK found in our cells. When these signal relay stations become activated, they stimulate the production of the MMP genes and other genes that further increase the inflammatory environment of the cartilage cells. They also turn on "suicide genes," which release toxic chemicals that kill the cartilage cell. The result is cartilage breakdown and osteoarthritis.

DIET AFFECTS CARTILAGE DESTRUCTION IN THE JOINTS

There is significant research to support the idea that the diet we eat influences the amount of cartilage degradation that occurs in our joints. It does this by increasing the activity of the genes in cartilage cells that breakdown cartilage. These genes code for such substances as MMP-13, ADAMTS-4, and 5-LOX.[7] As you recall, MMPs or matrix metalloproteinases are proteases which cleave cartilage. ADAMTS is a group of proteases, which like the MMPs breaks down cartilage. New research is identifying more active substances, called cytokines and **chemokines**, which are involved in the development of osteoarthritis.[8] The body's inflammation and production of AGEs is increased when we consume an unhealthy diet of saturated and trans fats, as well as sugar and other "empty-calorie" carbohydrates. These inflammatory products accumulate in our joints and cause cartilage damage.

GENE THERAPY

New research is isolating enzymes responsible for cartilage destruction and working backward to identify which genes in the DNA sequence produce them. In osteoarthritis, aggrecan is broken down by a group of enzymes called **aggrecanases**. They belong to the ADAMTS family of cartilage-degrading enzymes. ADAMTS-5 is one such aggrecanase enzyme.[9] Gene therapy uses chemical compounds that target the ADAMTS-5 gene and shut it down. This can be used as a strategy to control the progressive cartilage deterioration that occurs in osteoarthritis.

Another avenue in gene therapy research looks at transferring desirable genes to osteoarthritic cartilage cells, where they can offset the damage done by destructive genes.[10] These new genes would then code for compounds that build up the cartilage matrix, as well as compounds that inhibit its breakdown (such as IL-1Ra, discussed below).[11] For instance, it is known that the chemical compound IL-1 is very active in cartilage destruction, so research is focusing on transferring the gene that codes for the **IL-1 receptor antagonist (IL-1Ra)** into osteoarthritic cartilage cells.[12] This receptor would then block the affects of IL-1, thus helping to control the destructive phase of osteoarthritis. Genes are transferred into cells using a select group of "safe" viruses. As we recall, viruses are very common in causing human disease. For instance, the common cold is caused by a class of viruses known as **rhinoviruses**. The virus is a nonliving protein and

DNA unit that infects cells and becomes incorporated into our DNA. There they express their own DNA leading to disease. These specially engineered "safe" viruses are able to enter cartilage cells and transfer the human gene they carry to our DNA. In this way, a type of "gene surgery" is performed in which we can insert a missing or malfunctioning gene into an individual's DNA. In the case of our efforts to block IL-1, when the virus "infects" the cartilage cell it starts producing multiple copies of the IL-1 blocking agent. This goes to work in neutralizing the destructive effects of IL-1. As the technologies to effectively perform this type of "gene surgery" become more sophisticated, gene therapy will be an important medical treatment.

"Safe" viruses are virus particles that have been chemically modified so that they cannot infect a cell as they normally do. They can also produce a large number of duplicate viruses. The virus itself is inactive and poses no threat.

Another promising research endeavor is identifying markers for osteoarthritis that can be detected early in the course of the disease, offering hope of being able to alter its course.[13] Examples of such markers include small breakdown fragments of cartilage matrix called **cartilage oligomeric matrix protein (COMP)**. Another evolving marker is blood and urine **pentosidine**. Pentosidine is an advanced glycation endproduct that has been found to accumulate in joint cartilage in osteoarthritis, causing the yellowish appearance of old and degenerative cartilage.

PPAR RECEPTORS AND INFLAMMATION

New research is shedding light on how specific nutrients can be used to treat metabolic syndrome and insulin resistance. The development of metabolic syndrome in the body leads to increased production of fatty acids that circulate in the blood and increased TNF-alpha production. These in turn activate the NFkB signal relay intermediate and modify the insulin receptors in cells, resulting in insulin resistance. At the molecular level, metabolic syndrome can be treated by dietary and lifestyle modifications.[14] This is done through the activation of the PPAR in cells, which decrease inflammation.[15] Stimulation of PPAR-alpha receptors clears fatty acids from the blood.[16] Stimulation of the PPAR-gamma receptors leads to the formation of smaller fat cells, which are less inflamed.[17] As discussed earlier, it is the oversized fat cells in the waists of obese people that wreak all the havoc of inflammation and disease in their bodies. Beneficial nutrients that activate PPAR receptors include soy proteins, licorice, cinnamon, ginseng, and a number of beneficial antioxidant compounds found in plants. Soy plant estrogens have also been shown to improve blood sugar levels in the body. EPA, the active ingredient found in fish oils, acts through PPAR receptors to stimulate fat breakdown and to improve the sensitivity of insulin.

FIBRONECTIN FRAGMENTS

Another emerging area of research in osteoarthritis involves the study of **fibronectin fragments**.[18] These are important in triggering cartilage breakdown—acting to increase inflammatory cytokines and MMPs—and they are overproduced in osteoarthritis. Cartilage cells that are stimulated by fibronectin fragments act through the NFkB mediator to trigger increased inflammation in joints. Researchers are looking at methods to block NFkB and stimulate PPAR-alpha and PPAR-gamma receptors as strategies to fight osteoarthritis.

CONCLUSIONS

1. Gene therapy is an exciting new technology which transfers desirable genes into diseased cartilage cells to combat the osteoarthritic process.

2. Beneficial nutrients which stimulate PPAR receptors can be used to treat metabolic syndrome, insulin resistance, and are part of the nutritional armamentarium to combat osteoarthritis.

3. PPAR-alpha and PPAR-gamma receptor activation is a major way healthful nutrients lower inflammation in our bodies.

4. NFkB is an important communicator of our environment and our nutritional habits to our genes. It is the cellular mechanism by which the environment interacts with our genetic predispositions to lead to either health or disease.

5. Activation of PPAR receptors through good nutrition blocks the NFkB receptors, which is the culprit in triggering inflammatory pathways in the body.

14

Beneficial Nutrients for Joints

Osteoarthritis can be attacked by a number of nutritional approaches that have been shown to have the following beneficial effects:

1. Lowering systemic inflammation and oxidative stress
2. Promoting cartilage repair
3. Promoting proper hormonal balance
4. Directly affecting gene expression in cartilage cells
5. Lowering the formation of advanced glycation endproducts

VITAMINS AND MINERALS

A major cause of osteoarthritic cartilage damage is the generation of oxygen free radicals in joints as a result of increased oxidative stress. To combat this stress, our major detoxifying enzymes, such as catalase and glutathione peroxidase must be functioning properly. If they are malfunctioning or are overwhelmed because they are processing excessive amounts of toxins, they cannot properly maintain joint health. Vitamins and minerals are important because they act as helpers, or *cofactors*, for these detoxifying enzymes. Some of the most important vitamins and minerals needed to maintain optimum joint health are vitamin C, vitamin E, glutathione, selenium, and **beta-**

carotene. Glutathione peroxidase is one of the body's major detoxi-fying enzymes, and it is a free radical scavenger. For it to function nor-mally and rid the cell of harmful toxins, adequate levels of the impor-tant mineral selenium are needed in the diet. Zinc and copper are important helpers for the proper functioning of the important detoxi-fying enzyme, superoxide dismutase.

Sadly, the modern American diet is too low in essential fatty acids; essential minerals such as magnesium, zinc, and selenium; as well as vitamins and antioxidants. It is necessary, then, for most of us to sup-plement our diets with a daily intake of multiminerals and multivita-mins in order to maintain joint health. I will be discussing the use of supplements in greater detail in chapters 15 and 16, but some of the important ones for osteoarthritis include glucosamine; chondroitin; SAMe; EPA and DHA omega-3 fats found in fish oils; vitamins C, D, E, and B; alpha lipoic acid; and coenzyme Q10.

Deficiency of the B-complex vitamin **folate** (folic acid) is very common in the diets of people who do not eat large amounts of fruits and vegetables. Double-blind studies have shown that arthritic patients taking folate supplements along with anti-inflammatory medication had reduced pain compared to those taking anti-inflammatories alone.[1]

SNP DIFFERENCES IN THE GENES CAUSE SOME PEOPLE TO BE MORE SENSITIVE TO NUTRITIONAL DEFICIENCIES

Single nucleotide polymorphisms result in individuals whose enzyme systems are not as powerful as those of others, resulting in the devel-opment of diseases. In these susceptible people, the genes coding for certain detoxifying enzymes have SNP variations that lead to the for-mation of enzymes that are less functional and less able to interact with their helpers (usually vitamins or minerals).[2] These vitamin and mineral helpers must be obtained from the diet, so a diet that is lacking in these helpers will result in a malfunctioning of their detoxification enzymes. The SNP variations make the detoxification enzymes less able to interact with the vitamin and mineral helpers. Since we cannot do anything about the specific SNPs in our genetic code, the way to correct this is to give higher doses of the minerals and vitamins to compensate for the fact that the enzyme is not as efficient in interacting with them. By giving enough of the vitamin or mineral necessary for the enzyme to function normally, we can override the defect in the enzyme.[3] This is the rationale behind the recommendation of nutritional and genetic scientists to take more daily vitamins and minerals than what is normally recommended: these larger doses are needed to restore metabolic balance.

HIGH-ORAC FOODS FIGHT OXIDANT STRESS

An important way to pick good foods to eat is by looking at the **oxygen radical absorbent capacity (ORAC)** value of the food. ORAC refers to the fact that a food contains in it valuable antioxidants that are able to neutralize oxygen free radicals in the body. Examples of such foods include blueberries, green and other colorful vegetables, tomatoes containing the powerful antioxidant lycopene, and strawberries, among others. The higher the ORAC value, the better, because high-ORAC foods are the best at absorbing damaging free radicals in our cells. Foods with a high ORAC value have antioxidant and anti-inflammatory properties that promote good health. The average person in the United States eats 1,800 ORAC units per day. In people with degenerative diseases such as osteoarthritis, up to three or four times that amount is needed per day to neutralize excessive free radicals and other oxidants. High-ORAC foods include the colorful plants and vegetables that are full of antioxidants. For instance, one cup of blueberries has an ORAC value of 3,240 units, one-quarter teaspoon of cinnamon has 2,675 units, one apple has 300 units, and one green tea bag has 1,200 units.

NIACINAMIDE AND OSTEOARTHRITIS

In the 1930s and 1940s, Dr. William Kaufman was a pioneer in treating osteoarthritic patients with nutritional supplements. He reported good results in treating patients with large doses of **niacinamide**, a form of vitamin B_3. Niacinamide in large doses proved to have anti-inflammatory properties. Today we know that B-complex vitamins are important in decreasing inflammation in the body by lowering levels of homocysteine,[4] an inflammatory compound that has been shown to be as important—if not more so—as cholesterol in leading to heart attacks.

In 1996, researchers were able to validate Kaufman's results. In a double-blind, placebo-controlled study, niacinamide was given to patients for three months. The result was a decrease of the inflammatory blood substance **erythrocyte sedimentation rate (ESR)**, and patients who were already taking anti-inflammatory drugs were able to decrease the dosage taken.[5] ESR is a protein found in blood that is found to be increased in people who have elevated inflammation in their bodies. These patients were also shown to have improved mobility and function of their joints.

SHORT-TERM STUDIES DO NOT SHOW THE BENEFICIAL EFFECTS OF NUTRIENTS

When studying the effects of nutrients on diseases, it is important to treat patients for a long period of time in order to see positive effects. Because they change the basic underlying chemical imbalances that cause disease, nutrients must be given for long periods of time to be beneficial. Drugs, on the other hand, tend to act much more quickly, often requiring only minutes or hours to work. This characteristic of drugs makes them more favorable in showing positive results when used in short-term scientific studies. When looking at the effects of

nonsteroidal drugs versus the nutraceuticals chondroitin and glucosamine, which I will be discussing in chapter 15, research shows
that drugs relieve the pain of osteoarthritis much more quickly than
glucosamine and chondroitin. Glucosamine and chondroitin are two
natural substances that normally belong in our joint cartilage. They are
used to build new cartilage, and, because osteoarthritis results in cartilage being lost in the joints, researchers have found that supplementing them in the diet can improve the pain and other symptoms of
osteoarthritis. In a short-term study, about six to twelve weeks,
researchers may not be able to demonstrate a positive effect by glucosamine and chondroitin, because in that short interval they have not
yet shown their beneficial effects. They must be given for a long
time—often months to years—in order to reverse the damage of
osteoarthritis. While nonsteroidal drugs tend to show earlier positive
results than nutraceuticals in terms of pain relief, it is important to
realize that none of the drugs thus far developed to treat osteoarthritis
has ever been shown to alter the course of arthritis or to modify the
underlying chemical imbalances causing this disease. They only treat
the symptom: pain. In saying this, I do not want to minimize the pain
relief people have found using anti-inflammatory drugs through the
years: it has been considerable. The nutraceuticals I will be discussing,
on the other hand, have been scientifically shown in many cases to
heal and reverse osteoarthritis with *long-term use.*

Nutritional substances that have been traditionally used in the
treatment of osteoarthritis, and have shown benefit in pain relief and
decreasing inflammation, include Boswellic acids, topical capsaicin,
cetylmyristoleate (CMO), methysulfonylmethane (MSM), topical
menthol, phytodolor, SAMe (S-Adenosyl methionine), shark cartilage, stinging nettle, white willow, turmeric (found in **curcumin**), and
green tea bioflavonoids (antioxidants found in green tea). I will be discussing some of these in more detail in chapter 15.

FIGURE 14-1
WAYS TO COMBAT METABOLIC SYNDROME

1. **Eat nutritious food, avoiding sugar and "empty-calorie" foods**

2. **Lose weight, especially around the waist**

3. **Exercise, including aerobic and strength training**

4. **Take important nutritional supplements:**

   - **N-acetyl cysteine**

   - **Omega-3 fats (fish oils)**

   - **Coenzyme Q10**

   - **Chromium picolinate**

   - **Alpha lipoic acid**

   - **Acetyl-L-carnitine**

   - **Vitamin C**

   - **B-complex vitamins**

   - **Vitamin E**

DNA, NUTRITION, AND OXIDATIVE STRESS

Degenerative diseases such as osteoarthritis, which are caused by a highly inflammatory and oxidative stress environment, require optimal nutrition high in vitamins, minerals, and antioxidants. Researchers have shown that even small deficiencies in folate, vitamin B_{12}, niacin, and zinc result in an increase in spontaneous DNA defects. The DNA damage resulting from increased oxidative stress activates harmful genes and can lead to diseases such as cancer. The standard American diet, which is low in fruits and vegetables, leads to nutrient deficiencies that increase oxidative stress and promote the occurrence of degenerative diseases and cancer.

CONCLUSIONS

1. Recent research is showing how nutrients interact directly with our DNA and influence which genes are turned on and off. Nutrients are able to interact with cells and change their chemical and electrical states.

2. Inflammatory foods, which create an acidic cellular environment, activate the NFkB signal messenger, which then activates inflammatory genes and increases the overall inflammation in the body.

3. During states of increased oxidative stress, the body's defenses (in the form of the detoxifying enzymes and their vitamin and mineral helper cofactors) become overwhelmed and toxic free radicals accumulate.

4. Inadequate levels of vitamin C, E, and other antioxidant nutrients lead to such a state of increased oxidative stress, and are a risk factor in the development of degenerative diseases. Researchers have shown that people with higher intakes of vitamins C, E, and A had slower progression of osteoarthritis of their knee than did people not taking these antioxidants.

5. Vitamins and minerals act as important helpers (i.e., cofactors) for the important detoxification enzyme systems.

6. SNP variation of the detoxification enzymes requires that we obtain adequate levels of vitamins and minerals through our diet and with the use of supplements in order to optimize the function of the detox enzymes.

7. Important supplements for osteoarthritis include glucosamine; chondroitin; SAMe; EPA and DHA omega-3 fats found in fish oils; vitamins C, D, E, and B; alpha lipoic acid; and coenzyme Q10.

8. High ORAC foods such as berries and colorful vegetables absorb damaging free radicals in the body.

15

The Nutraceutical Arsenal Needed to Combat Osteoarthritis

O ur nutrition affects the proper functioning of our genes through a process called **epigenetics**. Epigenetics is a process by which certain genes are turned on and off in our DNA by the addition of methyl groups to the DNA sequence. These changes, which occur in our DNA because of our nutritional habits, surprisingly, can be passed on to our children. The ability of diet to alter our DNA highlights the important role the environment plays in influencing our genetic makeup. It also supports the importance of proper nutrition in preventing cancer and degenerative diseases, such as osteoarthritis, that are so prevalent today. The benefits of nutrition can be contrasted to drugs. None of the drugs currently employed in osteoarthritis has been shown to change the course of the disease.

The concept that nutritional and environmental factors can alter our DNA epigenetically, and that this change can be passed on to our future generations, is very important. This means that nutrition is much more important than previously thought in causing permanent changes to our DNA.

Good nutrition is powerful medicine, but it takes longer to show the positive effects of nutrients given to treat diseases when compared to drugs. Nutrients can be used in combinations to treat diseases. This additive effect is called **synergism**. In order to show the positive effect of nutrients in scientific experiments, it is important to design the experiments to look at the effects over a long period of time. Some of the studies that have been critical of the effectiveness of nutrients in treating diseases have been poorly designed. Some of these studies have been short term, with a small number of patients enrolled. In some cases, the studies were looking for other outcomes and coincidentally found that a nutrient did not have any effect. These studies were not designed to specifically test for the individual nutrient and are therefore not as trustworthy. The fact is that nutritional treatments work slowly because they act in combination with a number of other nutrients and environmental conditions to alter the body's chemistry over the long term. Studies to test the effectiveness of nutraceuticals must be designed with this in mind and be long-term studies with an appropriate endpoint and the appropriate choice of a time frame in which the effect is demonstrated.

SAMe AND OSTEOARTHRITIS

First discovered in 1952, SAMe is an important chemical produced in the body using the amino acid **methionine**. SAMe is a factor in many important enzymatic reactions in the body. These important chemical reactions, known as **methylation reactions**, are involved in many housekeeping and detoxification functions in the body. SAMe is important to joints because it has been shown to increase the synthesis of proteoglycans, the basic subunits that make up the three-dimensional cartilage matrix. SAMe also decreases the inflammatory response by decreasing the action of the gene that codes for the inflammatory compound TNF-alpha, a toxic cytokine involved in osteoarthritic cartilage destruction.

METHYLATION REACTIONS AND DETOXIFICATION

S-adenosylmethionine (SAMe) is a sulfur-containing compound involved in the important methylation reactions occurring in the body.[1] SAMe is formed from dietary methionine and choline, and some of it is directly manufactured by the body. Methionine is an **essential amino acid**, which means that the body cannot make it but must get it from the food we eat. Methionine is important in the detoxification enzyme systems of the body. It acts by being chemically modified in a process called methylation. In the process of detoxification, a toxic compound known as homocysteine is generated. Homocysteine has recently been implicated as a known risk factor for heart attacks. It is a toxic compound, and if it builds up in the bloodstream it leads to dangerous levels of inflammation. Homocysteine is cleared from the blood by being turned into the nontoxic methionine. For homocysteine to be eliminated, we must have adequate levels of vitamin B_{12} in our bodies.[2] This is because vitamin B_{12} acts as a helper for the enzyme which gets rid of homocysteine from our blood.

SCIENTIFIC STUDIES SUPPORT THE USE OF SAMe IN OSTEOARTHRITIS

In a double-blind study looking at how SAMe stacks up against the popular nonsteroidal anti-inflammatory drug Celebrex, people were given one of these two substances for sixteen weeks.[3] In the first month of the study, Celebrex showed a better reduction of arthritic symptoms, but by the second month there was no difference between the two groups.

In a subsequent SAMe clinical study, SAMe was shown to have a slower onset of action, but with equal results to anti-inflammatory medications at four weeks of treatment.[4] SAMe was also shown to stimulate the synthesis of new cartilage. These same researchers did a **meta-analysis**, which is a large study that combines the results of other studies. In this case, the results of twenty-two thousand patients treated with SAMe were reviewed, showing that SAMe was effective in the treatment of osteoarthritis.

A basic science study in which rabbits were given SAMe showed that it increased the cartilage thickness and the number of cartilage cells in these animals.[5] This study highlighted the cartilage-protective properties of SAMe.

Ninety-seven hip and knee osteoarthritis patients were studied for twenty-four months in multiple hospitals.[6] These patients were given 600 mg of SAMe daily for two weeks, followed by 400 mg daily for the rest of the two-year period. The SAMe was found to control osteoarthritic pain, and no side effects were observed at two years. SAMe also helped the depressive moods of osteoarthritic patients.

A double-blind clinical trial looking at the effectiveness of SAMe versus the nonsteroidal drug Indocin was carried out for four weeks.[7] In this study, SAMe was found to be just as effective as Indocin in improving the symptoms of arthritis.

In a double-blind, placebo-controlled clinical trial testing SAMe versus the nonsteroidal drug Piroxicam in knee osteoarthritis patients, researchers found both to be effective in pain relief and both to be well tolerated.[8] The advantage of SAMe was shown in that it had a **positive carryover effect**—that is, patients continued to show improvement for a number of months after the medicine had been stopped. This positive carryover effect is seen with nutraceuticals such as SAMe, but is not seen in drugs, which stop having any effect soon after their use is discontinued.

Another double-blind clinical trial compared SAMe with Motrin in thirty-six patients with knee and hip osteoarthritis. The researchers found equal improvement in all osteoarthritis symptoms in both these groups.[9]

B-COMPLEX VITAMINS ARE NEEDED TO LOWER HOMOCYSTEINE LEVELS AND INFLAMMATION IN THE BODY

The important enzyme **methylenetetrahydrofolate reductase (MTHFR)**, which eliminates the toxic homocysteine from our bodies, needs appropriate levels of B-complex vitamins in order to function properly.[10] As discussed earlier, SNPs (single nucleotide polymorphisms) are single subunit changes in a long string of subunits that make up a gene. New genetic research has shown that in some people, the gene coding for the MTHFR enzyme has an SNP that makes them hypersensitive to low B-complex vitamin levels in their diets. When these individuals do not consume enough B-complex vitamins, MTHFR does not function properly and is not able to neutralize and clear homocysteine from the blood. In these people, homocysteine builds up in the blood, predisposing them to heart disease. Research has shown that nutritional deficiencies in folate, vitamin B_{12}, and vitamin B_6 also conspire to decrease the proper elimination of homocysteine, resulting in increased inflammation in the body.[11] Elevation of homocysteine in the blood is seen in inflammatory and degenerative diseases.

A deficiency of B-complex vitamins has another detrimental effect in that it causes less cysteine to be produced, which is needed to form glutathione. **Glutathione** is an important helper in the detoxification enzyme system (glutathione peroxidase), which is needed to neutralize free radicals. Glutathione assists glutathione peroxidase to perform detoxification functions. In the absence of adequate levels of B-complex vitamins, oxygen free radicals are not appropriately eliminated from our cells, causing damage.

An experiment conducted on osteoarthritic mice, in which they were fed a blend of vitamins C, B, E, and A, and selenium, found that this combination of nutrients decreased osteoarthritis symptoms and the severity of the disease. Researchers also showed that animals taking this combination of nutrients were less likely to develop osteoarthritis—that is, the treatment prevented the disease from occurring. When they looked at the biochemistry of the cartilage cells in these animals, researchers found that their detoxification enzymes superoxide dismutase and glutathione peroxidase were increased in concentration. They concluded that the benefit of these vitamins in osteoarthritis was a result of their ability to increase the functioning of the antioxidative enzymes. This is why these nutrients are referred to as antioxidant nutrients.

OTHER NUTRIENTS AND OSTEOARTHRITIS

MSM

Methylsulfonylmethane (MSM) is a sulfur-containing substance found in fruits and vegetables. One double-blind, randomized clinical trial showed that people with knee osteoarthritis treated with MSM for three months had significantly increased function and decreased pain compared with those taking a placebo. Another recently published study looking at the ability of MSM to treat osteoarthritic knee pain and disability showed that MSM was very effective in controlling the symptoms of osteoarthritis.

CMO

Cetyl myristoleate (CMO) is beneficial in the treatment of osteoarthritis because it inhibits the COX and LOX enzymes that produce inflammatory compounds in the arachidonic acid pathway. In one randomized, controlled study it was found that CMO was beneficial in controlling the symptoms of knee osteoarthritis, with fewer side effects than nonsteroidal anti-inflammatory drugs.

Boron and Selenium

Two other nutrients that have been shown to have beneficial effects on osteoarthritis are boron and selenium. Research has shown an association between low boron levels and osteoarthritis. Boron is involved in the proper metabolism of calcium, which is needed to maintain strong bones. In areas of the world where boron intake is low, there is a seven-fold increase in osteoarthritis incidence compared to areas where boron intake is adequate.[12] In one experiment arthritic hips removed during surgery were studied for their boron content; they were found to contain half the boron content of normal hip bones.[13]

Selenium has been shown by scientific experiments to be important in maintaining healthy cartilage cells. In animal studies rats fed a low-selenium diet showed increased degeneration and malfunctioning of their cartilage.[14]

ASU: Avocado and Soybean Extracts

Avocado/soybean unsaponifiables (ASU) is a newly discovered substance that has been shown to be effective in treating osteoarthritis. ASU extracts are obtained from chemical processing of avocado and soybean oils. Recent research indicates that they have powerful anti-inflammatory effects. Antioxidant flavonoids contained in soy have been shown to decrease oxidation in cells. They also decrease C-reactive protein levels, which in turn decreases systemic inflammation.

Studies Show That ASU Has Beneficial Effects in Osteoarthritis

A number of researchers have studied the effects of ASU on osteoarthritis.[15] In one prospective, randomized, double-blind, placebo-controlled multicenter trial—the gold standard in research for generating reliable results—164 patients with osteoarthritis were treated.[16] A prospective study is one in which people are given a treatment and then are followed into the future to see how they respond to that treatment. The results indicated that the ASU group had significantly decreased pain and functional disability compared to the control group, which was not given the substance. This study also demonstrated a carryover effect in that the ASU group showed persistent beneficial effects even two months after treatment was discontinued. This positive carryover effect is often seen in nutraceuticals used to treat osteoarthritis and is one of the advantages they have over drugs, which do not have this effect.

In another experiment in which osteoarthritis was induced experimentally in animals, ASU showed a protective effect on cartilage by increasing the cartilage matrix produced and decreasing the amount of bone damage seen in osteoarthritic joints.[17] This study highlighted the disease-modifying benefit of ASU in improving the function and chemistry of the arthritic cartilage. Remember that none of the drugs currently used for osteoarthritis has any disease-modifying effect.

Researchers have shown that soy protein also improves osteoarthritis-associated symptoms.[18] Soy has been shown to increase concentrations of IGF-1—the compound that directly blocks the effects of the cartilage-degrading IL-1 cytokine—in the blood. An added benefit of soy is that it reduces the generation of glycoprotein fragments as cartilage is broken down. These fragments themselves are capable of generating further inflammation and cartilage destruction.

Antioxidants and Osteoarthritis

Research has shown that people given high-antioxidant diets experienced decreased inflammation in their bodies, and blood concentrations of inflammatory compounds were significantly decreased. Human cartilage cells that are exposed to an environment of high oxidative stress produce more damaging free radicals and have more damage to their DNA.[19] These cartilage cells also die prematurely. This is the underlying chemical process that perpetuates osteoarthritic damage in our joints.

Antioxidants, which are found in high concentrations in vegetables, are very important for proper detoxification in the body. Some of these key antioxidants include **lycopene, lutein, anthocyanidins,** and **xanthines**. As discussed previously, high-ORAC foods contain important antioxidants. These include **trans-resveratrol** in red wine, **polyphenols** in green tea, lycopene in tomatoes, and **bromelain** in pineapples. Berries, garlic, kale, and spinach also contain high antioxidants. Important anti-inflammatory spices, herbs, and fruits include turmeric, ginger, garlic, onion, cayenne, rosemary, parsley, and citrus fruits.

Trans-resveratrol in Red Wine

Trans-resveratrol, the active antioxidant ingredient in red wine, has been studied to determine its effects on osteoarthritis. In one study, researchers injected trans-resveratrol into the joints of arthritic rabbits, resulting in a decrease in cartilage destruction.[20] Another study demonstrated that healthy men who were given 30 g per day of red wine for four weeks had a 21 percent decrease in C-reactive protein (the inflammatory protein found in blood) and a decrease in overall inflammation in their bodies.[21]

Trans-resveratrol, which is also found in the skin of red grapes, has powerful anti-inflammatory and anticlotting effects. Studies have shown that this antioxidant protects obese mice from developing obesity-related illnesses such as diabetes and heart disease. It is also powerful in activating genes that combat the effects of aging: it turns on genes that produce enzymes known as **sirtuins**, which have beneficial effects in lowering disease rates and extending life in mice. More research into the benefits of this important antioxidant is under way.

MMP GENE INHIBITORS: GREEN TEA AND TRITERPENOIDS FIGHT OSTEOARTHRITIS

Recent research has shown that green tea antioxidants, called **bioflavonoids** reduce the levels of cartilage-degrading MMPs.[22] They do this by blocking the signal intermediate NFkB, and they also directly block the genes that code for MMPs. Experiments have been done in which the inflammatory cytokine IL-1 was used to activate NFkB. When EGCG, the active chemical substance found in green tea, was given, it was found to block the ability of NFkB to move into the nucleus and activate cartilage breakdown genes.

Steroids are also potent MMP gene inhibitors, as are **retinoids**, which are vitamin A derivatives. The problem with steroids in treating osteoarthritis is that their long-term use can actually accelerate cartilage damage. Steroids were thought to be a cure for arthritis when first discovered back in the 1950s because of their powerful actions in improving arthritis pain and inflammation. Now, as a result of their side effects, their use is limited in the treatment of osteoarthritis.

Triterpenoids are a class of plant compounds that have been shown to inhibit the genes that overproduce MMPs in osteoarthritis.[23] They include oleanolic acid and ursolic acid, and have been isolated from commonly known herbs such as ginseng, eucalyptus, and rosemary. Clinical studies have shown that these substances are effective in improving arthritis symptoms. Oleanolic acid has been shown in rat and mice experiments to effectively counteract chemically induced experimental osteoarthritis. Triterpenoids also decrease the LOX and COX enzymes involved in the production of inflammatory prostaglandins and leukotrienes in the arachidonic acid pathway. In this manner, triterpenoids act similar to nonsteroidal anti-inflammatory drugs such as Motrin, Naprosyn, and Celebrex, which are useful in osteoarthritis because they are potent COX enzyme inhibitors.

Green Tea Flavonoids

Green tea contains important antioxidant substances that belong to the general class of compounds known in the plant world as **flavonoids**.[24] Flavonoids are the chemical substances in vegetables that give them their colorful appearance. It is important to eat a diet full of colorful vegetables, because these colors are an indication that the vegetables have a high concentration of healthful flavonoids. The two most important flavonoids in the fight against osteoarthritis are the **soy isoflavones** found in ASU and the catechins found in high concentrations in green tea.

Research has shown that catechins from green tea, when added to osteoarthritic cartilage cells in scientific experiments, stopped the breakdown of cartilage seen in osteoarthritis.[25] Green tea was thus shown to be cartilage protective and nontoxic in this experiment. In another experiment, **green tea catechins** were shown to block the production of cartilage-degrading MMPs, thus slowing down cartilage destruction.

Other Antioxidants

N-acetylcysteine is an important antioxidant that blocks the destructive action of the RAGE receptors.[26] Recall that cartilage cells contain the RAGE receptors on their surface. When we eat a diet high in sugar, our bodies develop chronically elevated blood sugar levels, which trigger the formation of the toxic advanced glycation endproducts. When the AGEs enter our joints, they target the RAGE receptors and activate them. This union of AGE and RAGE triggers the activation of the signal relay intermediate NFkB, which then turns on destructive cartilage genes. NAC works by blocking the RAGE-AGE-induced triggering of NFkB, thus preventing the breakdown of cartilage. Furthermore, NAC is the chemical used to build the important free radical scavenger glutathione,[27] which is used to make glutathione peroxidase, a very important detoxification enzyme. Thus, by taking NAC as a nutritional supplement in our diets, we support the detoxification enzymes in our body that rid our cells of damage-causing toxins.[28]

S-allylcysteine, found in garlic, is a natural antioxidant that blocks the formation of AGEs.[29] By including this in our diet, we can lower the production of these damaging sugar-coated proteins, which are so detrimental to our joint cartilage.

Vitamin C and Osteoarthritis

Vitamin C Helps Cartilage Cells Build Cartilage

Vitamin C has a number of beneficial roles in the building and maintenance of cartilage. It stimulates cartilage production and is a cofactor in important chemical reactions used by cartilage cells to form new cartilage. Without vitamin C, old cartilage would not be replaced by healthy, young cartilage and joint destruction would quickly result.

Vitamin C Is a Powerful Antioxidant

Vitamin C is a very important antioxidant and free radical scavenger and neutralizer.[30] It is important in offsetting the harmful effects of the increased blood free fatty acids found in metabolic syndrome and insulin resistance. It does this by blocking the inflammatory effects of oxygen free radicals and nitric oxide, which are generated by these increased fatty acids. It protects the cell membrane fats from undergoing harmful oxidizing reactions that increase oxidative stress in cells. Increased inflammation and increased free radical damage in joints damages cell membrane lipids. This damage is detected in the blood in the form of increased oxidized fats. When the cell membranes become damaged, the cells do not function properly. This is because cell membranes are responsible for keeping harmful substances from entering the cell and are important in transmitting chemical signals to the cell DNA. Thus, a malfunction of the cell membrane is comparable to the malfunctioning of a television and radio tower, with the resultant loss of electronic communication. It is also analogous to losing the protective barrier that encloses radioactive material in a nuclear reactor plant: the result would be flooding of the environment with dangerous and toxic waste.

Vitamin C is also important in decreasing the formation of AGEs, with the assistance of another important antioxidant compound, alpha lipoic acid (ALA). In this capacity, vitamin C decreases the quantity of AGEs available to stimulate the RAGE receptors found on the surface of cartilage cells from triggering cartilage breakdown. Research has shown that increased oxidative stress in the body reduces vitamin C blood levels. Studies have shown that low blood vitamin C levels were strongly associated with increased death in the elderly.[31] The large Framingham study (1996) showed that people taking large amounts of vitamin C had a threefold reduction in the risk of osteoarthritis progression.[32] X-rays of osteoarthritic patients found that vitamin C decreased cartilage loss and also decreased the progression of osteoarthritis. Similar effects were observed with the antioxidant vitamins E and beta-carotene in this study.

Another study looked at the effects of vitamin C on cartilage metabolism by studying guinea pig cartilage samples.[33] The researchers found that vitamin C stimulated the production of collagen and aggrecan—the two most important three-dimensional structures that make up cartilage—in joints.

In a randomized, placebo-controlled trial involving 133 patients with knee osteoarthritis, researchers showed that people treated with 1 g of calcium ascorbate (containing 898 g of vitamin C) had significantly decreased pain compared to those who were given a placebo.[34]

In a basic research study, when vitamin C was added to cartilage cells that had been previously exposed to an environment of high oxidative stress, it was shown to increase their life span.[35]

Vitamin E and Osteoarthritis

The Scientific Studies Showing the Benefit of Vitamin E in Osteoarthritis

Researchers have looked at how cartilage cells respond to oxygen free radicals when they are exposed to the caustic substance hydrogen peroxide. They have shown that hydrogen peroxide causes oxidative stress and damage to cartilage cells.[36] This results in the three-dimensional cartilage structure breaking down in the classic form of osteoarthritis. When vitamin E was added to the cartilage cells, the researchers observed less fat oxidation and protein damage consistent with oxidative stress, resulting in the reversal of oxidative damage to cartilage cells.

In another study, researchers experimentally induced osteoarthritis in the knees of rats by injecting hydrogen peroxide into their joints.[37] This duplicated the environment of increased oxidative stress that is seen in the body as a result of poor nutrition and environmental toxins. When they added vitamin E to this toxic environment, they found that it prevented the development of osteoarthritis.

In a clinical study involving people with osteoarthritis, a researcher looked at fifty osteoarthritic patients who were treated with 400 IU (international units) of vitamin E per day for six weeks versus those who were given a placebo.[38] This double-blind, placebo-controlled clinical trial showed that vitamin E was better than placebo in pain relief, and it was also shown to lower the need for pain medications in these patients.

Another double-blind study looked at how vitamin E compared to the anti-inflammatory drug Diclofenac when given for three weeks to patients with osteoarthritis.[39] The researchers concluded that vitamin E and the anti-inflammatory drug had equal ability to decrease knee swelling and pain.

Vitamin D and Osteoarthritis

Vitamin D is important for the proper maintenance of bone.[40] Vitamin D stimulates cartilage cells to synthesize the components needed to build cartilage. It is widely known that vitamin D is important in the prevention of osteoporosis, and we have discussed how joint bone is an important player in the development of osteoarthritis. Thus vitamin D plays a key role in osteoarthritis. Low levels of vitamin D in the body—as a result of poor intake of vitamin D, low exposure to sunlight, and the "epidemic" use of sunscreen—have been implicated in weakening our bones and predisposing us to osteoarthritis. Although sunscreen is important in preventing skin cancer, it is also important that we obtain some direct sunlight every day (up to a half hour), because this helps form vitamin D in our skin. People who live in northern climates and who stay indoors much are often found to be vitamin D deficient because they do not get enough sunlight each day.

The large Framingham study showed that people with low amounts of vitamin D in their diets had a threefold increase in the risk of progression of osteoarthritis compared to those those consuming large amounts of vitamin D.[41]

A scientific study looking at how vitamin D levels in the blood correlated with the progression of hip osteoarthritis on x-rays[42] showed that low blood levels of vitamin D were associated with progressive hip joint space narrowing, which is a cardinal sign of progressive joint deterioration and progressive osteoarthritic destruction.

Fish Oils and Osteoarthritis

Fish oils contain the important omega-3 fatty acids discussed earlier. The modern American diet has a low ratio of omega-3 to omega-6 fats, which is unhealthy. Omega-3s are found in fish oils, nuts, flaxseed, and canola oil. The omega-6 fats are mostly found in corn oil, sunflower oil, and meat products. As discussed previously, high omega-3 has strong anti-inflammatory properties; omega-6 fats, on the other hand, are processed through the arachidonic acid pathway to form inflammatory prostaglandins. Both omega-3 and omega-6 fats are important, but the ratio is tilted toward omega-6 fats as a result of their excessive consumption in modern diets.

Studies of the effects of fish oil supplements in osteoarthritis have been positive. In one study fish oil supplements were given along with Motrin to patients.[43] Researchers found that pain relief was higher when fish oils and Motrin were given together as opposed to when Motrin was used alone.

Other researchers have shown that omega-3 fatty acids decrease breakdown of cartilage in osteoarthritis.[44] Omega-3s were found to decrease the production of cartilage-degrading enzymes and inflammatory compounds in cartilage. They blocked the action of the degrading compound IL-1 and also decreased the action of the LOX and COX enzymes in the arachidonic acid pathway. As we recall, anti-inflammatory drugs such as Motrin also exert their pain-relieving effects by blocking the LOX and COX pathways, which form inflammatory prostaglandins.

ALPHA LIPOIC ACID, ALCAR, AND OSTEOARTHRITIS

Why Alpha Lipoic Acid Is an Important Nutraceutical in Osteoarthritis

Alpha lipoic acid acts as a cofactor for important enzymes in the energy-producing powerhouses of our cells, the mitochondria. ALA has been shown to be important in regulating the levels of antioxidants such as vitamin C, vitamin E, and the free radical scavenger glutathione. ALA recycles these antioxidants so they can be reused in the cell to fight oxidative stress. In this role, ALA effectively increases the concentration of these important nutrients in the cell.

ALA further combats the formation of the toxic advanced glycation endproducts. It has beneficial effects in improving insulin sensitivity and lowering blood glucose, which results in decrease in the formation of AGEs in the body.[45] It also attacks the RAGE receptor found on the surface of cartilage cells, blocking the activation of this inflammatory receptor. By blocking RAGE, ALA acts to protect cartilage and prevent cartilage breakdown. In research studies in which oxidative stress is produced in cells by adding hydrogen peroxide, the resultant cellular damage is countered by the addition of ALA.

ALCAR Is a Powerful Antioxidant

Scientific experiments showed that the detrimental effects of aging were reversed in aging rats when they were fed food supplemented with acetyl-L-carnitine and alpha lipoic acid antioxidants.[46] Memory skills, as well as overall energy and activity levels in these "old" rats were improved.[47] The researchers showed that less oxidative stress was seen in these rats when given ALCAR, with decreased oxidative damage seen in their blood fats and proteins, as well as the DNA in their cells. In essence, these rats got younger when given these supplements!

In another study, researchers reported that the function of the energy-producing mitochondria in cells was increased when ALCAR[48] and ALA[49] were given. Experiments in rats supplemented with these two nutrients showed that they had improved agility, improved ability to walk, and increased energy production.

CHROMIUM PICOLINATE IS BENEFICIAL IN DECREASING AGEs

Chromium picolinate is important in regulating blood sugar levels and in promoting the proper functioning of insulin in the body. Scientific experiments in obese rats treated with chromium have shown

---

FIGURE 15-1
SUPPLEMENTS THAT DECREASE CARTILAGE CELL
ENLARGEMENT AND HELP FIGHT OSTEOARTHRITIS

The following substances have been shown by research to block the formation of advanced glycation endproducts and are thus useful in the prevention of "plump" cartilage cells, which are responsible for triggering the development of osteoarthritis:

carnosine
ALCAR
chromium picolinate
alpha lipoic acid
l-arginine

---

improvement in their blood sugar levels. This is because chromium improves the transport of glucose from the blood into cells in organs such as muscles and the liver. This clears the blood of glucose and prevents the formation of AGEs. Thus, chromium decreases oxidative stress and lowers free radical formation in our organs. Researchers studying the effects of chromium on animals showed that animals which were fed chromium picolinate lived one-third longer than other animals. When chromium was tested in humans, it was shown to lead to less obesity by decreasing fat accumulation in the body.

GLUCOSAMINE AND CHONDROITIN: WHAT IS THE BOTTOM LINE?

Glucosamine and chondroitin are two important nutraceuticals in the arsenal of fighting osteoarthritis.[50] My purpose here is to review the largest and most well-conducted studies, including the largest randomized clinical trials, that support the use of these two powerful substances. These two substances must be more regularly and enthusiastically supported by doctors when discussing the various treatment options with patients suffering from osteoarthritis. Studies have shown that chondroitin and glucosamine combinations provide anti-inflammatory effects by decreasing the production of inflammatory prostaglandins through the blocking of the COX-2 gene. The COX-2 gene codes for the COX-2 enzyme that is responsible for the formation of inflammatory prostaglandins. As we have learned, too much arachidonic acid in the diet leads to activation of COX-2 in the arachidonic acid pathway and to the production of excessive inflammation in the body. Chondroitin delivers a double-punch by also blocking the gene that codes for the enzyme, which is responsible for generating the oxidative and inflammatory substance nitric oxide, which has been previously discussed.

GLUCOSAMINE SCIENTIFIC STUDY RESULTS

The long-term effects of glucosamine sulfate on osteoarthritis progression were studied by scientists using a randomized, placebo-controlled clinical study involving 212 people with knee osteoarthritis.[51] Patients in the study group were given 1,500 mg of glucosamine and those in the control group were given a placebo every day for three years. These researchers looked at the appearance of x-rays taken of the knees of these patients one year and three years after the beginning of the study. In the placebo group, 106 patients were shown to have progressive joint space narrowing of 0.31 mm. Joint space narrowing is an indication of the cartilage deteriorating in the joint. X-rays are able to visualize only the two bones, the femur and tibia, that make up the knee joint. The cartilage that makes up the cushion in the joint is seen as "empty space" on the x-ray, and it is referred to as the joint space. As osteoarthritis progresses the joint space becomes narrower as the cartilage deteriorates and the top femur bone starts to grind on the bottom tibial bone. This is the process referred to as "bone-on-bone" osteoarthritis and is an indication that the disease is very advanced. In this experiment, contrary to the placebo group, the glucosamine group showed no joint space narrowing. Patients did not experience any further cartilage loss while they were given the glucosamine. The glucosamine group also showed improvement in their pain, stiffness, and swelling at three years, while the placebo group was found to have worsened symptoms. This study highlights the ability of glucosamine in halting the disease progress of osteoarthritis, thus being an effective disease-modifying substance. It is effective in also improving the pain and swelling seen in osteoarthritis. The other important aspect of glucosamine demonstrated by this study is that for it to be effective, it must be used for a long period of time (in this case, one to three years).

Studies that are unable to show the effects of glucosamine are often short-duration studies. Researchers looked at the effects of glucosamine by studying the response of patients treated for two months with 500 mg per day.[52] This study failed to show positive results, but it was limited by its short duration and the low dose of glucosamine used.

Another group of researchers did a three-year randomized, placebo-controlled, double-blind study in 202 patients with knee osteoarthritis; half were given 1,500 mg glucosamine sulfate each day and the other half were given a placebo.[53] The symptoms of osteoarthritis were improved in the glucosamine group. In the control group, joint space narrowing on x-rays was shown to get worse, while the joint space was stabilized in the glucosamine group, showing that the progression of arthritis was stopped.

A study conducted with 205 people examined the results of patients given a twelve-week course of 1,500 mg glucosamine per day versus those given a placebo.[54] This study failed to show beneficial effects by glucosamine.

A double-blind study of 178 patients who were given a four-week course of 1,500 mg per day of glucosamine or 1,200 mg of ibuprofen (Motrin) found that glucosamine was more effective than ibuprofen in improving osteoarthritic symptoms, and that glucosamine was also better tolerated.[55] Short-term studies are not optimal for study of neutraceuticals, but they can show positive results, as this study does.

A multicenter, randomized, placebo-controlled, double-blind

study involved 252 osteoarthritic patients.[56] Glucosamine was given at 500 mg three times per day in the study group, and placebo was given in the control group. These researchers showed that glucosamine was statistically superior to placebo in relieving osteoarthritis pain, in increasing the distance these patients were able to walk, and in improving their daily overall function.

Another multicenter, randomized, placebo-controlled, double-blind study looked at 155 knee osteoarthritic patients. Half of these patients were given 400 mg shots of glucosamine twice a week for six weeks, while the other half were given a placebo.[57] Researchers were able to show that glucosamine had statistically better effect on osteoarthritis than did placebo in relieving osteoarthritis pain, increasing their walking distance with no pain, and improving their overall function.

A 2004 randomized, double-blind, placebo-controlled study enrolled 118 osteoarthritic patients.[58] These patients were split into four groups receiving one of four treatments: group 1 received glucosamine at a dose of 500 mg per day for three weeks, group 2 received the nutraceutical MSM 500 mg per day for twelve weeks, group 3 received glucosamine 500 mg and MSM 500 mg together per day, and group 4 received a placebo for twelve weeks. Patients in groups 1, 2, and 3 showed improvement in their osteoarthritis over group 4. Of special interest is that group 3, which received glucosamine and MSM together, showed the highest amount of pain relief and greater anti-inflammation benefits. This study highlights the important concept that nutraceuticals work well together and have additive effects when given in combinations.

A meta-analysis looking at the combined results of fifteen other glucosamine studies found that in this large number of patients, glucosamine was an effective nutraceutical in the treatment of osteoarthritis.[59]

Conclusions of the Glucosamine Studies

Overall, most of the large glucosamine studies (more than 100 people) with long-term follow-up (greater than six months) have shown that glucosamine is an effective disease-modifying nutraceutical and also an effective pain reliever in people with osteoarthritis. The limited glucosamine trials that did not show a positive effect on osteoarthritis have certain characteristics in common. A major weakness of these negative trials was the short duration of the study period. Others enrolled patients with very advanced osteoarthritis or gave them lower doses of glucosamine. Because glucosamine modifies the disease slowly, when studied in patients with advanced disease or when given for a short period of time, it is not likely to be shown effective. Glucosamine is effective in protecting the cartilage from progressive damage due to osteoarthritis. This cartilage-protective effect occurs with long-term use and may not show up in short-term trials that look for quick onset of action and quick pain relief. Because of glucosamine's disease-modifying properties, it has the best chance of working if used early in the onset of osteoarthritis and taken for a long period of time.

CHONDROITIN SCIENTIFIC STUDY RESULTS

Chondroitin has been found to be effective in the treatment of osteoarthritis in at least eleven randomized, controlled studies. Long-term clinical studies have shown that chondroitin stops the deterioration of arthritic joints and prevents further collapse of the joint. Chondroitin works by providing the building blocks to make hyaluronic acid and proteoglycans, which form the three-dimensional structure of joint cartilage. It also reduces the breakdown of collagen, which forms the "backbone" of cartilage, and reduces cartilage cell death. It has important actions in blocking the cartilage-degrading MMP enzymes, and it decreases inflammation buildup in joints by blocking the action

FIGURE 15-2
GLUCOSAMINE AND CHONDROITIN STUDIES

	Results Positive (yes) Negative (no)	Length of Study	No. of Patients Studied
Glucosamine Studies:			
J. Y. Reginster et al.	Yes	36 mos.	212
J. P. Rindone et al.	No	2 mos.	49
K. Pavelka et al.	Yes	36 mos.	202
T. E. McAlindon et al.	No	3 mos.	205
G. X. Giu et al.	Yes	4 weeks	178
A. Reichelt et al.	Yes	6 weeks	155
W. Noack et al.	Yes	4 weeks	252
P. R. Usha et al.	Yes	3 mos.	118
T. E. McAlindon et al. (15-trial meta-analysis 2000)	Yes	> 4 weeks	?
Chondroitin Studies:			
T. Conrozier	Yes	12 mos.	104
B. Mazieres et al.	Yes	5 mos.	120
B. A. Michel et al.	Yes	24 mos.	300
P. Morreale et al.	Yes	6 mos.	146
B. F. Leeb et al. (7-trial meta-analysis)	Yes	> 4 mos.	372

2. Vitamin deficiency in the body allows for the buildup of toxic substances such as free radicals, leading to the malfunctioning of important toxin-eliminating enzymes. Vitamin B-complex deficiency leads to increased inflammation by increasing homocysteine levels in the body and also by decreasing the body's ability to fight free radicals.

3. Our nutrition is able to cause changes in our DNA, which we are able to pass on to our children.

4. MSM has been shown by scientific studies to be effective in the treatment of osteoarthritis. It can be often found in a triple combination with glucosamine and chondroitin, which are two other effective nutraceuticals.

5. Cetyl myristofleate (CMO) has similar action to nonsteroidal anti-inflammatory drugs with lower side effects.

6. The current research supports the use of soybean and avocado extracts in fighting the pain and inflammation of osteoarthritis. Studies have shown that ASU has cartilage-building properties and can increase formation of the structural backbone of cartilage, collagen. ASUs block the detrimental effects of IL-1 and can lower the production of the cartilage-degrading MMPs. ASU has the potential to modify disease, thus improving the cartilage condition in osteoarthritis.

7. New research supports the use of vitamin C in the treatment of osteoarthritic patients. Experiments using vitamin C in arthritic patients have shown that vitamin C must be taken in doses of up to 1 to 2 grams per day in order to have optimal antioxidant effect.

8. Vitamin E enhances cartilage cell growth and protects cartilage cells against free radical damage. A number of double-blind, placebo-controlled studies have shown that vitamin E intake of 400 IU for six weeks is significantly superior to placebo in relieving pain in people with osteoarthritis. The conclusion is that vitamin E is a beneficial supplement in the nutraceutical arsenal for the treatment of osteoarthritis.

9. The scientific evidence thus collected supports the role of vitamin D as an effective nutrient in osteoarthritis by slowing its progression. More double-blind clinical studies are needed to further elucidate the effects of this important bone and cartilage nutrient.

10. Omega-3 fatty acids found in fish oils are effective nutraceuticals in maintaining overall joint health and decreasing the inflammatory response seen in the cartilage destruction of osteoarthritis.

11. ALCAR and ALA lower oxidative stress and improve mitochondrial function in cells. They make the generation of energy from food more efficient. You can think of ALCAR and ALA as similar to carburetor-cleaning fluid, which, when added to gasoline, makes the burning of the fuel more effi-

cient and "cleaner." These two important supplements also combat the formation of AGEs, which are so detrimental to cartilage and which are a result of unhealthy eating and the development of metabolic syndrome and insulin resistance. *ALCAR and ALA are important neutraceuticals in the treatment of osteoarthritis.*

12. When using nutritional treatments to treat osteoarthritis, we must focus on combining a number of nutrients in order to increase their effectiveness. Nutrients are able to complement each other and show additional benefits when combined. An example of this is the combination of glucosamine, chondroitin, and methylsulfonylmethane (MSM) in the same tablet. Nutritional treatment of disease involves having the proper balance of nutrients over a long period of time in order to alter the course of disease. In the case of osteoarthritis, nutraceuticals have been shown to have disease-modifying properties drugs do not have. This ability to improve a disease state, as opposed to merely treating symptoms, gives nutraceuticals an edge over drugs.

13. Nutraceuticals promote cartilage repair and directly activate and deactivate genes in cartilage cells. On the other hand, drugs that are currently used to treat osteoarthritis have not been shown to have disease-modifying properties; they are instead aimed at reducing symptoms rather than affecting the underlying causes of the disease. Nutritional treatments have a solid scientific basis and should be incorporated in mainstream medical practice for the benefit of those patients who are suffering from osteoarthritis.

14. Chondroitin has been shown in a number of prospective, double-blind, placebo-controlled studies performed at multiple hospitals to be effective in the treatment of osteoarthritis. It reduces pain, improves joint mobility, improves function, and reduces the need for drugs such as nonsteroidal anti-inflammatories. One important characteristic of chondroitin is

that it continues to provide improved function and pain relief even when it has been stopped. This is not the case with non-steroidal anti-inflammatory drugs, which quickly wash out of the system once they have been stopped.

15. Glucosamine and chondroitin are two important nutraceuticals that have been shown to treat osteoarthritic pain effectively and also to possess disease-modifying effects that lead to reversal of the arthritic process in joints.

16. Glucosamine and chondroitin work slowly, and at least twelve weeks of treatment is necessary to see effects. Studies have shown that they have long-term beneficial effects even after treatment has been stopped. Long-term x-ray studies have documented that they rebuild cartilage.

17. Glucosamine and chondroitin are aptly termed *slow-acting disease-modifying agents* in the treatment of osteoarthritis.

18. The combination of glucosamine and chondroitin has been shown to decrease inflammation by blocking the production of prostaglandins and blocking activation of the RAGE receptors involved in cartilage breakdown pathways.

19. In spite of multiple studies illustrating their effectiveness, these nutraceuticals have received only a lukewarm reception by the medical community thus far.

Part 4

MY DIETARY RECOMMENDATIONS FOR OSTEOARTHRITIS

16

Dietary Recommendations in Osteoarthritis for the New Millennium

As discussed earlier, poor nutrition leads to increased inflammation and oxidative stress in the body. It causes metabolic imbalances that deteriorate joints, leading to the development of osteoarthritis. In previous chapters I have presented the most recent scientific findings that support this theory. In this chapter I will discuss my dietary recommendations for the treatment of osteoarthritis, which are based on the latest scientific evidence.

Traditionally, doctors have treated osteoarthritis with drugs. There is currently a renewed interest among scientists in using naturally occurring compounds to treat diseases such as osteoarthritis. These substances have been shown in both double-blind clinical trials as well as personal experience by doctors and patients to be beneficial and to have few, if any, side effects. It is important to also understand that, as of 2008, only nutritional substances have been shown in scientific studies to slow down and reverse osteoarthritis. Laboratory-manufactured drugs have never been shown to have any positive effect on the underlying causes of osteoarthritis; they only relieve pain. In fact, laboratory-manufactured steroids and nonsteroidal anti-inflammatory drugs have been shown to actually accelerate the progression of osteoarthritis when used for long periods of time. Think about it: the most commonly prescribed drugs by doctors not only do not help reverse or cure the disease, but they may actually be harmful with long-term use.

UNHEALTHY DIETS INCREASE INFLAMMATION

A number of scientific studies have shown that people who have good diets consisting of anti-inflammatory fats and healthful vegetables have lower inflammation in their bodies.[1] Inflammation is measured by the blood levels of the proteins ESR and CRP, which are increased in states of high inflammation. The current epidemics of obesity and metabolic syndrome are a result of unhealthy diets that increase the inflammation in the body. These same poor dietary habits and obesity increase the generation of free radicals and degrading chemicals in our joint cartilage. The recent explosion of osteoarthritis that physicians have seen over the last twenty years is fueled by our unhealthy eating habits. The result is that surgical replacement of arthritic joints—at younger and younger ages—has skyrocketed in the last fifteen years.

The two most dangerous conditions in our bodies predisposing us to the increased degeneration of our organs, including our joints, are increased blood sugar levels and increased levels of unhealthy fats. Americans consume more refined sugar per year than almost any other nation. The consumption of synthetic trans fats is ruining our health. In 2007 the city of New York passed laws designed to limit the use of synthetic trans fats by restaurants. This trend will undoubtedly be followed by other cities. The chronic state of high blood sugar in our bodies as a result of our heavy consumption of soft drinks and other junk food generates increased inflammation and increased oxidative stress. These detrimental effects have been scientifically proven. The sugar accumulating in the bloodstream has many detrimental effects, leading to the development of diabetes, nerve damage, and cartilage damage. As discussed earlier, elevated blood sugar destroys cartilage by creating sugar-coated proteins called AGEs. These act to turn on genes in cartilage cells that code for cartilage-destructive substances. In this way, our diet affects the function of our genes. AGEs also bind to cartilage, weakening it and turning it a sickly yellowish color.

Recommendation #1: Limit your intake of refined sugars, soft drinks, candy bars, and other sweets. Eliminate unhealthy trans fats from your diet completely. Trans fats are listed on food packaging as partially hydrogenated oils and are contained in cake mixes, potato chips, and other nonperishable foods. Limit the consumption of saturated fats, found in red meats, and increase the intake of healthful nuts, monounsaturated olive oil, and omega-3 fats found in coldwater fish and flaxseed. Poor nutrition leads to a vicious cycle of increased inflammation and "rusting" in our bodies. This has led to the explosion of obesity and unhealthy blood sugar and cholesterol levels that is fueling the new epidemic of cartilage deterioration and osteoarthritis development.

My experience in the treatment of osteoarthritis patients in my own clinical practice is that they are very interested in how nutrition affects their disease. People are tired of being prescribed drugs, with all their side effects, to treat their joint pain. They are looking for new information and fresh approaches to their disease. Traditionally, complementary and alternative medicines have been in high demand among osteoarthritic patients. When I see patients in my practice in the early stages of osteoarthritis, I use the nutritional recommendations I have listed in this chapter to arrest and reverse the progression of this disease. As I have shown, a number of quality scientific studies support the use of nutritional interventions in osteoarthritis.

DO WE REALLY NEED VITAMIN AND MINERAL SUPPLEMENTS?

I am often asked in my own practice, "Doctor, if I have a healthy diet, why do I need extra supplements?" The answer to this question is that we are constantly bombarded by many man-made chemical substances, such as environmental pollution, pesticides, and unhealthy food preservatives. We need to supplement our diets with vitamins and minerals in order to ward off disease. Eating a good diet is the keystone to good health. Vitamins and minerals taken in supplement form complement a good diet and are important because of genetic variations between individuals in handling the many pollutants we come in contact with. As you recall from previous chapters, our bodies detoxify the many thousands of chemicals they come into contact by using detoxification enzyme systems. Vitamins and minerals aid these systems, helping them do their job efficiently. The more toxic our environment is and the worse our diets are, the more important it is to supplement our diets with vitamins and minerals.

Scientific studies have also shown that the body's ability to detoxify itself differs from person to person. Some people are able to rid of toxins better than others. These people naturally require less nutritional support in the form of vitamins and minerals. The problem is that currently there is no test to accurately determine whether an individual is a good detoxifier. The genetic testing required is not yet sophisticated enough to do this. The ability to detoxify is determined by our genetic makeup. Recent genetic studies are beginning to show that single nucleotide polymorphisms, which are small variations in the structure of key genes among individuals, control our detoxifying ability. New research has also shown that larger doses of vitamins and minerals than what has been traditionally recommended by doctors are required to restore the function of the often inefficient and overwhelmed detoxification enzyme systems and to help prevent the development of degenerative disease.

Recommendation #2: We need to maintain a low fasting blood sugar level (75–90 mg %) and a weight within the parameters of a body mass index of less that 25 and body fat less than 16–18 percent. The blood sugar level is the concentration of sugar in the blood, which is measured after fasting for eight hours. BMI is calculated by using the formula below. (Note: weight is in pounds and height is in inches.)

BMI Formula:

$$\frac{Wt \times 703}{Ht \times Ht} = BMI$$

BMI Results:

25–29 is overweight

30–39 is obese

> 40 is extremely obese

Low blood sugar and low body fat content will go a long way in guaranteeing that we do not have dangerously high levels of inflammation in our bodies.

NUTRITIONAL SUBSTANCES HELP STOP AND REVERSE THE PROGRESSION OF OSTEOARTHRITIS

Nutrients that have been shown by the latest research to be effective in stopping and reversing the progression of osteoarthritis are called nutraceuticals. Unlike laboratory-manufactured drugs, which have many side effects, these substances are normally found both in nature and in our bodies and are not toxic, as drugs are. When using nutrients to combat osteoarthritis, it is important to use combinations of these nutrients that work well together. We need to find the proper balance of beneficial nutrients and to use them for a long period of time. Unlike drugs, which are fast acting, nutrients work slowly to exert their beneficial effects.

Recommendation #3: The following nutraceuticals can be used to decrease the damage of osteoarthritis in joint cartilage. These can be found in most health food stores, and I recommend using brand names made by reputable companies.

alpha lipoic acid	600 mg twice a day
coenzyme Q10	60 mg twice a day
L-carnitine	1,000 mg twice a day
N-acetylcysteine	1,000 mg twice a day
acetyl-L-carnitine (ALCAR)	500–400 mg per day
miacinamide	250 mg four times per day
DHA (fish oils)	2 grams per day
EPA (fish oils)	1 gram per day
selenium	200 mcg per day
glutathione	300–600 mg per day
vitamin C	1,000–2,000 mg per day
vitamin D	400–1,200 IU per day
vitamin E	400–800 IU per day

In order to support our energy-producing mitochondria and to lower inflammatory proteins in our blood while lowering oxidative stress, we need to have optimum levels of B-complex vitamins.

Recommendation #4: The following B-complex vitamins are useful for the treatment of osteoarthritis. B-complex vitamins are important in supporting the detoxification enzymes and also in decreasing oxidative stress in cartilage cells.

vitamin B_6	25 mcg per day
vitamin B_{12}	1,000 mcg per day
folic acid	800 mcg per day

Recommendation #5: I recommend the daily use of the quadruple combination of the following four supplements in people with osteoarthritis or with a strong family history of the disease in order to control pain and also prevent progressive collapse of the joint:

glucosamine HCl	1,500 mg per day
chondroitin	1,200 mg per day

MSM   1,500 mg per day

SAMe   200–600 mg per day

WHAT IS THE BEST DIET FOR OSTEOARTHRITIS?

The scientific evidence outlined in this book supports diet as a very important determinant of the inflammatory status of the body.[2] A diet loaded with sugar leads to the development of pre-diabetes and to organ damage. Eventually, a heavy consumption of sugar in the diet leads to the development of diabetes, with its many life-altering complications. Some estimates predict that up to one-quarter of children born in the year 2000 are destined to develop diabetes unless their diets are drastically changed in the next decade. This is a very alarming statistic. Our unhealthy diets are fueling the development of type 2 diabetes, heart disease, and atherosclerosis.

Recommendation #6: Osteoarthritis patients should adhere to the Mediterranean diet, outlined in chapter 8. This diet is loaded with good fats and is low in sugar. It is high in healthy fats, such as olive oil and omega-3s. It has been shown to lower blood cholesterol and triglyceride levels, increase the blood levels of "good fats," and decrease the overall inflammatory state of the body.

WHY IS WEIGHT LOSS IMPORTANT IN THE TREATMENT OF OSTEOARTHRITIS?

In traditional medicine, weight loss is thought to improve osteoarthritis symptoms by decreasing the weight placed on our joints and thus lowering stress-related damage to the cartilage. As shown in this book, obesity is also related to osteoarthritis in complex biochemical pathways that involve increased inflammation and increased oxidative stress. While it is true that weight loss and the maintenance of an optimum weight level of BMI less than 25 lowers the mechanical stresses on our joints, it more importantly lowers inflammation and decreases the oxidative stress that predispose us to osteoarthritis.[3]

Recommendation #7: There is very good scientific evidence that weight loss improves osteoarthritis symptoms in overweight patients.[4] Research has also shown that a combination of moderate weight loss and moderate exercise (such as twenty to thirty minutes per day, five days per week of walking or aerobics) improve the symptoms of osteoarthritis and decrease joint pain more than weight loss or exercise alone do.[5] I recommend weight training and aerobic exercises three to five times per week and maintaining a BMI below 25. The dietary recommendations I have made in this chapter are based on a concept known as **evidence-based medicine**. Evidence-based medicine refers to the practice of medicine that is supported by basic clinical research, not just traditional, anecdotal treatments or physician preference. More good-quality research studies need to be done in the future to elucidate the benefits of nutraceuticals in the treatment of diseases.

HOW TO PREVENT THE DEVELOPMENT OF OSTEOARTHRITIS

The best way to avoid developing degenerative joint disease is by adopting the following strategies:

- Maintain an optimal body weight with BMI of 25 or less.
- Eat a diet low in sugar and high in omega-3 fats.
- Maintain physical fitness. Aerobic exercise should be done at least twenty to thirty minutes per day, for three to four days per week. Supplement this with two to three days per week of muscle strengthening.
- Avoid the development of excess inflammation and oxidative

stress in the body by eating healthy colorful vegetables, lean proteins, and supplementing your diet with vitamins, minerals, and other nutrients.

- Use prophylactic nutritional supplements, such as glucosamine, chondroitin, MSM, and SAMe, if you have a strong family history of osteoarthritis.
- Maintain a healthy alkaline pH in your body by eliminating unhealthy trans fats, refined sugars, white flour, soft drinks, and juices.
- Minimize high-impact and contact sports after the age of forty to avoid repetitive joint injuries.
- Maintain a waist size of less than 36 inches for men and 30 inches for women.
- Maintain a normal blood sugar level to avoid developing insulin resistance and diabetes.

These preventive measures are more powerful than drugs in treating and preventing osteoarthritis.

Part 5

IT IS TIME FOR A PARADIGM SHIFT IN MEDICINE

17
Why We Need a Paradigm Shift in Medicine

We need a paradigm shift in medicine.[1] We need to attack degenerative diseases, such as osteoarthritis, with more holistic treatments that will be safer and more cost-effective in the long run. Expensive drugs, high-tech surgical procedures, and other invasive treatments are major factors that have led to our expensive and increasingly unaffordable healthcare system.

Paradigm shifts have occurred in the history of medicine and science in the past. Today many doctors and lay people realize that it is necessary to change the way medicine is practiced. It is time for medical practitioners to change the way new scientific evidence and discoveries are viewed and implemented. The concept of *paradigm shift* was popularized by Thomas Kuhn, a physicist and philosopher of science, in his book *The Structure of Scientific Revolutions*,[2] in which he explains that scientific progress occurs as old beliefs are challenged by new ways of looking at problems. He describes science as having long stable periods during which most scientists hold the same core beliefs and look at scientific data through the same "colored lenses." These periods are interrupted by paradigm shifts, during which scientists learn new ways to think about old problems by questioning long-held beliefs. This builds a momentum of dissent in the scientific community, and eventually the "old" paradigm is replaced by a new one.

Paradigm shift becomes necessary in science as more research is done in a certain discipline and new knowledge is accumulated, giving rise to inconsistencies in that these findings cannot be reconciled with the old paradigm. Scientists working in the old paradigm cannot deal with the new scientific evidence and tend to discard it. *We are currently in such a paradigm shift in terms of the new advancements being made in the understanding of chronic and degenerative diseases.*

We need to incorporate the basic science discoveries in nutrition and genetics more effectively into our healthcare delivery system in order to halt the epidemics of obesity and degenerative joint disease in this country. In many major medical centers today, some of the busiest surgeons are the ones performing weight loss surgery, which was practically unheard of ten or fifteen years ago. This fact in itself is very telling of our current epidemic obesity.

We must also stop focusing on outdated nineteenth- and twentieth-century principles of a single disease with a single magic-bullet cure. This approach will not work for the complex diseases of the twenty-first century. These diseases, such as dysfunction in our metabolism and the degeneration of our organs, require a deeper understanding of what exactly is going wrong in the body. Drugs designed in the lab should not be our main weapon in treating degenerative diseases. We need to stop praying at the altar of pharmaceutical "wonder drugs" and instead adapt the safer alternatives described in this book for medical use. The public is inundated by drug advertisements in the media. Physicians have bought into the belief that laboratory-designed drugs are superior to any other method of fighting disease. The truth is that a holistic approach that integrates basic scientific knowledge from current nutrition and genetics research in fighting osteoarthritis is more effective in treating the early stages of this disease, preventing its progression, and ultimately reversing its course. As I have shown, there is a large body of nutritional and genetic research that needs to be effectively incorporated into the everyday treatment of patients.

Organized medicine does not recognize the benefits of proper nutrition in fighting specific diseases. Vitamins, minerals, and nutraceuticals are also powerful in producing a disease-free metabolic state. Basic scientific research in nutrition and biochemistry is continuing to elucidate the powerful ways nutrition can fight degenerative disease. The problem is that the public is not being properly educated by the current medical system about these new discoveries in nutritional genetics, the nutritional treatment of degenerative diseases, and the dangers of runaway inflammation and metabolic syndrome in the body.

Many economic pressures prevent physicians from adopting a more holistic approach when treating patients. As a result of the pressure in modern medicine to see large numbers of patients each day, doctors are often rushed through the visits and can only address serious issues as they occur. They are focused on prescribing drugs to treat health conditions. Discussions of alternative treatments are difficut to undertake in the limited time of an office visit. Thus some restructuring is needed in the way patients are screened for diseases and on how they are educated about their health. In an integrated health system, this can happen through patient seminars and by group visits of multiple patients with the same condition where education can be interactive. Restructuring healthcare to address chronic diseases is important so that diseases can be diagnosed early and treated more effectively. Also, because doctors are becoming more specialized, they are more focused on their own narrow fields of interest and can lose perspective on their patients' overall health. As a result of these and other factors, many physicians do not fulfill their mission as health educators. I believe the public is "hungry" for a more holistic and integrated approach to their health. They want doctors to help them stay healthy, not just treat illnesses as they develop. They do not go to see a doctor simply to have their symptoms treated with a prescription of an expensive and often potentially toxic pharmaceutical drug. This is one reason why many prescriptions written by overworked physicians go unfilled. This is also one of the reasons that chiropractic and alternative medical approaches are so popular: These practitioners tend to be more holistic—more "hands-on"—and they spend more time with their patients than traditional medical doctors do.

What about the great advances that have been made in medicine over the last half century? When we look critically at this issue, other than the advances made in surgical treatments and early detection, the medical approach to degenerative disease has failed to effectively treat diseases such as osteoarthritis. Osteoarthritic patients are primarily treated with pain-relieving drugs until it is time to perform joint surgery. This is the current "state-of-the art" treatment of this disease.

Until physicians become better advocates for maintaining the health of their patients, rather than reactively fighting disease whenever it crops up, medicine will fall short of fulfilling its mission. By the time disease becomes apparent—with the development of symptoms of pain and swelling—significant damage has already occurred in the body. New research into nutrition and genetics will allow us to diagnose and treat the early metabolic and chemical imbalances that occur in the body before they develop into serious diseases. This research makes possible the early diagnosis and treatment of the imbalances that result from poor nutrition, exposure to environmental toxins, and stress. Furthermore, we are only beginning to learn how genetic predispositions, manifested in the form of gene single nucleotide polymorphisms, interact with the environment to determine the state of an individual's health.

As a result of the epidemics of obesity and metabolic syndrome, which accelerate osteoarthritis development, the typical osteoarthritic patient presents at a younger age than in the past. That person is usually first treated by a family doctor with pain medications, nonsteroidal anti-inflammatory drugs, and physical therapy. When these treatments no longer prove effective, the patient is referred to an orthopedic surgeon, who may treat with cortisone and other injections before finally resorting to surgery. As can be seen from the above scenario, the major—often invasive—treatments currently offered to patients treat only the symptoms. No new treatments have been developed in the last ten to fifteen years for these patients—even though basic scientific research has rapidly increased our knowledge at the cellular and genetic level during this time.

THE CURRENT MEDICAL PARADIGM TREATS DEGENERATIVE DISEASES WITH DRUGS

Our current medical paradigm emphasizes the use of drugs in treating degenerative diseases such as osteoarthritis. Because of this mindset, we have not made many strides in incorporating the new scientific research findings regarding inflammation and the interaction of nutrition with our genes in our medical treatments. More clinical research is needed to validate the many basic science and animal research findings that relate to nutrition, genetics, and inflammation. There has been little interest in doing this type of research in the nutritional treatment of disease. The reason for this lack of interest is that the search for new drugs (which is the "holy grail" of scientific research) has overshadowed these efforts. Part of the reason for this overemphasis on drugs is that the pharmaceutical industry provides much of the funding for clinical trials. The industry's emphasis is on promoting research that develops new, patentable drugs, even though nutritional treatments and nutraceuticals are much cheaper and safer alternatives.

WHAT ARE THE WEAKNESSES OF THE CURRENT MEDICAL PARADIGM?

Medicine's focus is not in preventing disease, but rather in treating disease once it has occurred. This "acute-care" medicine is not well equipped to deal with the complex, chronic diseases of the twenty-first century, because when a patient presents with a disease, the chemical imbalances at the cellular and organ levels have often gone undetected for a long time. These cell and chemical imbalances are not best treated with drugs, which are often designed to treat only symptoms and not the underlying chemical imbalance. While our basic scientific knowledge of diseases has continued to grow in the last decade, the translation of this new knowledge into clinical practice is very slow. This is the case in the treatment of osteoarthritis.

Another weakness in our system is that its emphasis on "acute-care" does not address well the best ways to attack chronic, degenerative diseases. Our system is excessively focused on crisis intervention rather than prevention. It is focused on finding a single "magic-bullet cure" for diseases, which was more appropriate when dealing with infectious diseases of the last century. A single drug can be effective in treating a single infectious disease, such as tuberculosis or staph infection, but the degenerative diseases of the twenty-first century are not going to be solved using this mentality.

Our current system lacks an integrated and holistic approach needed in addressing the chemical imbalances that cause chronic disease. It is focused on physician subspecialization and on crisis intervention, rather than on disease prevention.

Medicine rewards conformity rather than innovation. This conformity of modern medicine is best highlighted by the widely used "standardized treatment guidelines," which sacrifice the biochemical individuality of the patient and undermine the clinical judgment of the doctor. They are being pushed by medical societies and insurance companies as a panacea in improving healthcare outcomes and controlling costs. Clinical guidelines erroneously assume that all patients are alike and they all need the same drugs or the same surgical treatment. Genetic research, on the other hand, is showing that there is large genetic variability among individuals in how they respond to their environment, stress, and drugs. These differences are expressed in the form of single nucleotide polymorphisms among individuals. This genetic variability demands a more personalized approach to each patient, and requires that physicians be able to integrate many sources of information in order to individualize treatment.

DEFINING HIGH-QUALITY MEDICINE

Quality in medicine has been defined as the combination of a positive clinical outcome (for example, curing a disease) and the value to the consumer of the care delivered.[3] When we analyze the quality of medicine provided today, a number of shortcomings become apparent. In terms of both our diagnostic abilities and our surgical treatments, we are very advanced. We have state-of-the-art diagnostic equipment such as MRIs, CT scans, and PET scans, which increase our diagnostic accuracy and help save lives.

But when we look at the quality of treatments offered to patients, modern medicine starts to show its weaknesses. Physicians prescribe many drugs, which can have serious side effects, often for less-than-life-threatening conditions. Very often, the side effects of these drugs are more problematic than the symptoms they were prescribed to treat. These are referred to as "lifestyle drugs," and are used to enhance normal function rather than save lives or fight disease. These include Viagra, as well as numerous duplications of drugs by pharmaceutical companies in an effort to gain market share. Elderly patients taking multiple drugs often experience significant illness or even death from those drugs, even though they were properly prescribed and appropriately taken.

As stated previously, a weakness in modern medicine affecting quality is that it does not effectively incorporate new scientific advances into clinical practice in a timely manner. It also lacks an integrated approach to healthcare delivery. Healthcare is often fragmented, with tests and drugs being duplicated by multiple healthcare providers a patient sees, and heavily influenced by the threat of litigation.

Modern medicine is not good at appropriately identifying and treating the early chemical imbalances that occur in the body as a result of poor nutrition, stress, and environmental pollution. These often go undetected, eventually leading to full-blown disease. When the disease is finally apparent, the treating doctor is "behind the eight ball" and often resorts to controlling pain and other symptoms with the use of expensive and potentially toxic drugs. Because doctors are busy "putting out the fires" in their patients presenting with diseases, they do not often have the time to appropriately counsel their patients on proper nutrition, avoidance of dangerous habits, prevention of disease, and the benefits of aerobic exercise and strength training.

In conclusion, because medicine does not treat chronic diseases in an integrated way, but instead treats only the symptoms of disease as they arise, the current medical system is not well equipped to antici-pate the development of diseases and stop the early chemical imbal-ances in the body that will eventually lead to full-blown disease. By treating diseases when they present at later stages, when multiple symptoms and organs are malfunctioning, is quite costly in terms of dollars spent. This is one of the reasons why the United States, even though it boasts the largest per capita spending on healthcare in the world, ranks below the top in the overall health and life expectancy.

A PARADIGM SHIFT IS NEEDED IN MODERN MEDICINE

A paradigm shift is needed in modern medicine. This is needed to address the epidemics of obesity, degenerative disease, and the detri-mental effects of poor nutrition. Many people don't realize that we have an epidemic of malnutrition in this country. When people think of malnutrition they think of starving and emaciated children in Africa. What is not widely understood is that, even though they are overweight, obese people in this country are also malnourished because the many calories they consume have very poor nutritional value and are loaded with toxic food additives and preservatives.

The old paradigm doctors are working with calls for the use of drugs in treating degenerative diseases such as osteoarthritis. Drugs worked well in the old paradigm of a single "magic-bullet" killing a single "foreign invader," as seen in infectious diseases. They are not sufficient though to address the complex conditions of metabolic syndrome, obesity, and inflammation. *We are now entering a crisis stage in medical science: a turning point in which the existing disease paradigm cannot adequately solve the epidemic health conditions of our time.* In the case of osteoarthritis, except for surgical treatments, which have shown great advancements in the last twenty years, we have much to learn in the prevention and medical treatment of this disease.

The new genetic revolution, with the unraveling of the mysteries of the nearly one hundred thousand human genes by the Human Genome Project, is heralding a new era in medicine in which we will be able to better identify and treat chronic diseases. New knowledge has accumulated showing that nutrition has powerful effects on our genes. This new field of **nutrigenomics** is exploding with new discoveries that will be useful in treating the underlying biochemical and genetic imbalances involved in degenerative diseases such as osteoarthritis.

In order to make real progress in curing the degenerative diseases of our time, we must find new ways to interpret and implement basic scientific discoveries. Currently, new knowledge is not being integrated into clinical practice because it does not fit the old paradigm regarding when disease occurs in the body and how to best treat it. Conflict exists because scientists look at the same set of data from a different point of view. There is much controversy regarding the causes and effects of common medical conditions: Are heart attacks caused primarily by high cholesterol levels, or are they primarily an inflammatory disease, with cholesterol playing a secondary role? Is degenerative joint disease in osteoarthritis best treated by drugs, or by nutritional and nutraceutical interventions? These examples highlight the conflicts that exist in modern medicine, in which clinical problems are looked at differently by physicians functioning under the old paradigm than they are by those working in the new, emerging paradigm.

OUR HEALTHCARE SYSTEM IS IN CRISIS

Our healthcare system consumes a large portion of our gross national product, and its high expense is threatening our economic growth and prosperity. Furthermore, it does not adequately address the epidemic conditions of obesity, cancer, metabolic syndrome, and degenerative disease. Even though we spend a great deal of money on healthcare, we are not winning the battle in these chronic conditions. There are currently about 20 million people suffering from diabetes in our country. About one in seven people can be classified as pre-diabeteic, with elevated blood insulin levels and blood sugar levels. Increased inflammation and metabolic syndrome are rampant, and the current generation of children born in the United States is the first generation in history expected to have a lower life expectancy than their parents. These statistics are frightening and are fueling a debate among scientists regarding the best ways to implement healthcare changes to fight chronic diseases. Throwing more money in research that looks for answers using the old paradigm will not likely be successful in addressing these epidemic conditions.

Dr. David Eddy, known as one of the leaders of evidence-based medicine, has proposed that *only 15 to 25 percent of what doctors do in current medical practice is backed by "hard" scientific evidence.*[4] Eddy further suggests that in our high-tech healthcare system—estimated to cost about $2 trillion per year—there is no evidence that our current treatments are really any better than other, cheaper alternatives. My point here is that even though in the current medical paradigm, drugs and surgical treatments are significantly valued above nutritional treatments, as has been shown by Dr. Eddy, only a small portion (15–25 percent) of what doctors do in medical practice has been thoroughly scientifically studied and been found to be the most effective treatment. A paradigm shift of how doctors approach diseases is warranted, because I believe that there is enough scientific evidence proving the benefits of nutrition in treating and preventing disease.

ETHICS AND GENETIC INDIVIDUALITY

Finally, ethical principles must guide a move toward medical treatment of patients that respects each individual's genetic uniqueness. New research is proving the genetic individuality among people, and this must be incorporated into the ways we deliver healthcare. A disturbing trend is the idea that medical care can become standardized. The standardization of medical care is a popular concept proposed by think tanks and medical societies, which propose creating an "assembly-line" management of patients in which they are "processed" in large healthcare centers and are given generic treatments based on the use of popular clinical-practice guidelines. This "cookbook" approach is not supported by the new genetic research that is elegantly showing how the genetic individuality interacts with people's environment and nutrition in causing disease. Generic, "one-size-fits-all" treatment approaches—as practiced in the prescription of drugs, in which all patients are given a standardized dose of a drug—are not supported by these new and emerging scientific discoveries.

Part 6

NEW GENETIC FIELDS THAT WILL LEAD TO ANSWERS FOR OSTEOARTHRITIS

18
Looking to the Future

We are only just beginning to decode and understand the human genome. The DNA technology advancements that form the basis of the science of genomics include polymerase chain reaction technology and the development of **automated DNA sequencers**. These are technologies that can process large amounts of DNA material looking for a specific gene.

Gene chip technology is an evolving field that combines computer microprocessor chip technology and genetic engineering biology. **Gene chips** are built using a process known as *photolithography*, which is the same process used to manufacture microprocessors. The power of gene chips lies in the fact that they are packed with genetic probes that bind to DNA, similar to the way transistors are packed into a computer chip.[1] One chip can pack up to four hundred thousand individual probes, which are applied to decoding the human genetic code, which includes about one hundred thousand known genes. The ability in the last decade to perform **high-speed gene sequencing** using computers has fueled the speed at which new genetic information about human disease is gathered. Gene chip technology has the potential to speed up the change in the way diseases are treated, and even holds the possibility of reclassifying diseases as a result of our improved understanding of their causes. Currently in medicine, we often treat only the symptoms of diseases because we are unable to identify their underlying root causes. In the future we will be able to run a sample of cells through a gene chip scanner and analyze an individual's predisposition to certain diseases and what treatments we should use to treat and even prevent disease.

The emergence of these new genetic technologies also highlights the ability of our genes to interact and even be shaped by our environment and our nutritional state. In the old paradigm, genes are looked at as fixed DNA sequences that seal our fate with regard to the development of certain diseases. The new paradigm that is emerging through gene research is that of **biologic potentiality**. This refers to the idea that genes confer a potential that can be dynamically altered by environmental factors such as nutrition. This concept is central to nutrigenomics, which studies the ability of nutrition to directly talk to our genes and affect their action.[2]

NUTRIGENOMICS

Nutrigenomics is an emerging field aimed at unlocking the mechanisms by which nutrition is able to directly alter the function and expression of our genes.[3] Nutrients stimulate the activation of genes so that they produce hormones, enzymes, and other biologically active substances that influence our health. Much of this book has been concerned with discussing these substances as they relate to osteoarthritis. People have genetic variability, and that is why different people respond to nutritional and other environmental stimuli differently. For instance, researchers have shown that a diet low in the beneficial omega-3 fats is associated with a strong inflammatory cell environment in people with specific SNPs in the gene coding for the enzyme arachidonate 5-lipoxygenase.[4] In individuals possessing this particular SNP variation, a dietary insufficiency of omega-3 fats can have detrimental consequences that are not seen in people with a different SNP variation in that gene.

The power of nutrigenomics lies in the ability of medicine in the future to identify those people who are at high risk for developing a disease. Those individuals can then be treated with specific nutritional and pharmaceutical agents to prevent disease.[5] These advances will involve use of gene chip analysis and the technology of gene sequencing. Large segments of DNA containing many genes will be studied simultaneously to determine how the expression and activation of certain genes is affected by nutritional and other treatments. In osteoarthritis, gene chip analysis has shown that osteoarthritic cartilage cells show increased activation of genes that code for inflammatory and degrading cytokines compared to normal cells. These also include the increased expression of MMPs, which break down cartilage. Future studies with gene chips will be able to detect which genes are turned off and on in healthy versus diseased cartilage cells. Once these are identified, treatments can be developed that will turn on "good" genes while blocking the effects of inflammatory and cartilage degrading genes.

GENE THERAPY

Another promising field in the treatment of osteoarthritis is that of gene therapy.[6] Gene therapy research in arthritis has focused on IL-1 and other inflammatory compounds that are overproduced in the joints of persons with osteoarthritis. The blocking of IL-1 will be beneficial in preventing the joint destruction associated with arthritis. Special viruses, called "safe" viruses, have been genetically engineered to carry a gene in their own DNA that codes for a substance that blocks IL-1. That substance, known as IL-1 receptor antagonist, blocks the IL-1 by preventing it from stimulating its receptor in cartilage cells.

NUTRIGENETICS

Nutrigenetics is a related field that looks at how different nutrients affect our genes. The single nucleotide polymorphisms in our genes determine how we respond to different diets. SNPs have been discovered when genes taken from different individuals are analyzed using techniques such as the ones discussed above. Genes, which normally contain about three thousand DNA base pairs, have been shown to vary in only one base pair between different individuals. Certain SNPs can have a dramatic effect on how an individual responds to certain drugs, nutritional substances, or other chemical triggers. These SNP differences are the reason some people respond well to a drug while others experience terrible side effects.

A technique known as **high-throughput genotyping** can be used to study the effects of diet and specific nutrients on people possessing different genetic variations. One of the most well-studied SNPs is that of the enzyme MTHFR. This is an important enzyme that must function well in order to clear the inflammatory substance homocysteine from our blood. When individuals with a small change in the DNA sequence coding for this gene are subjected to a diet low in folate (a B-complex vitamin), they experience a significant and detrimental elevation in their blood homocysteine levels.[7] A diet low in B-complex vitamins can predispose these individuals to increased inflammation and the development of heart disease. Another well-known SNP is that of the PPAR-gamma receptor. In this case, a particular SNP variant predisposes people to developing increased blood insulin levels when that individual is given a highly inflammatory diet.[8]

Nutrition not only controls the action of our genes, it further acts in attaching to our DNA and causing it to function differently. This effect, known as an epigenetic effect, as previously discussed, is inheritable and can be passed on to our children. This epigenetic change is an important way in which our DNA is altered by the foods we eat and the environmental toxins we are exposed to. Thus, poor nutrition not only affects our genes in the present, but it also results in long-lasting changes in the DNA that we will pass on to our children.

PHARMACOGENOMICS

Pharmacogenomics is an emerging field that studies how an individual's unique genetic makeup relates to his or her ability to respond to, process, and eliminate drugs from the body. In this field, genetic engineering techniques are used to test a patient's blood in order to determine the optimal drug dose for that person and whether the drug should be given at all to that person. A drop of a patient's blood is placed on a gene chip, which can be tested to profile that person's interaction with the drug. For instance, one can examine the level of functioning of the important detoxification enzyme systems. As we recall from previous chapters, a person's detoxification systems may become overwhelmed when they are exposed to unhealthy food and other environmental toxins. That individual may not be able to effectively clear a drug from their system, allowing for the buildup of the drug and the development of unwanted side effects. Determinations can also be made from this genetic analysis as to what the optimal dose of the drug should be for that person. In the future, we will be able to respect a person's genetic individuality, rather than prescribing a standardized dose to everybody.

PROTEOMICS

Proteomics is the study of the interactions of proteins, which are the products of the action of our genes.[9] Genes code for proteins, and proteins then exert their biologic effects and act as the building blocks for our bodies. This field has great potential to aid in treating osteoarthritis because it can be used to identify early biomarkers for osteoarthritis before joint damage has occurred. Biomarkers can put us "ahead of the curve" by allowing us to predict a patient's risk of developing the disease before the onset of symptoms.[10] While there are about one hundred thousand genes in the human DNA, there are more than 1 million different proteins in the body that interact in complex ways. The technologies involved in studying large groups of proteins include those of **mass spectrometry, electron microscopy, electrophoresis**, and chip-related experiments. With these techniques, proteins that are unique to osteoarthritic patients can be identified by mass spectrometry and **two-dimensional electrophoresis**. Their potential as useful biomarkers, as well as their specific roles in the disease process, can be further studied in this way.

METABOLOMICS

Metabolomics is the study of how nutrients affect metabolic changes, which can be studied through the emerging technologies of **high-resolution nuclear magnetic resonance imaging** (commonly known as MRI or NMR).[11] In metabolomics, large groups of proteins can be studied simultaneously in order to shed new light into their interactions.[12] For instance, with the use of NMR, analysis is being done of the different effects on our metabolism of a variety of nutritional treatments.[13] Using this technology, the effects of nutraceuticals on our internal body chemistry can be studied.[14] Metabolomics and the use of NMR will be beneficial in unraveling these complex interactions. Using chemical pattern recognition, NMR is already being used to differentiate between disease states and normal states, as in the case of people suffering from cardiovascular disease and multiple sclerosis.

SOME THOUGHTS ABOUT THE FUTURE OF THE MEDICAL TREATMENT OF OSTEOARTHRITIS AND WHAT MUST BE DONE DIFFERENTLY

The nutritional strategies and healthy habits outlined in this book are more powerful than any laboratory-designed drug in treating and preventing osteoarthritis. Medicine's successes in saving lives by the early diagnosis of diseases, such as cancer, and "heroic" surgical procedures, such as joint replacement and brain surgery, have received a large amount of media attention. Similar advancements have not been made in treating and preventing the major chronic and degenerative diseases. This is because medicine's current way of attacking chronic diseases such as osteoarthritis with the use of drugs is flawed. Drugs have many unwanted side effects and are very costly. Furthermore, they do nothing to address the underlying causes of osteoarthritis. Why, then, are they so commonly used? This can be answered by realizing that medical doctors function under a set of beliefs and prejudices that have been reinforced through their extensive education. This is what is referred to as a paradigm.

In the current medical paradigm, physicians are trained to only treat the symptoms of osteoarthritis, with the use of anti-inflammatory drugs, painkillers, and steroid injections. Physicians must adopt a more holistic and integrative approach in treating osteoarthritis by incorporating the many new and exciting scientific discoveries of nutritional science and genetics outlined in this book. There exists a lag in medicine between the time basic science knowledge becomes available and when these concepts are incorporated into a doctor's everyday practice in treating disease. This is the case in the treatment of osteoarthritis, where new research in nutrition and genetics has not been appropriately included in the doctor's armamentarium to fight this disease. Unfortunately, physicians spend too much time writing prescriptions for drugs to treat the symptoms of diseases, rather than addressing their underlying causes. This results in patients—often the elderly—taking an excessive number of drugs that often have serious side effects.

Nutrition influences our genes and our hormonal state in powerful ways that translate to either good or bad health, depending on the choices we make. Proper nutrition is good medicine! Organized medicine must adopt the scientific discoveries of nutritional science and incorporate them into clinical practice in order to fight osteoarthritis more effectively and relieve the pain and suffering of its victims.

CONCLUSION

Proteomics, genomics, and metabolomics have great potential in the field of nutritional science and osteoarthritis research. These and other discoveries will give us the ability to study interactions of nutrients and inflammatory disease compounds at the molecular level and to determine their effects on our genes and cartilage. These newly emerging technologies provide great hope for unraveling the many debilitating diseases of our time. Overall, a more holistic approach is needed in approaching diseases such as osteoarthritis that will better incorporate new basic scientific findings into clinical practice in order to treat and eventually cure them.

Appendix
List of Inflammatory Compounds

advanced glycation endproducts (AGEs): Sugar-coated proteins formed by excess blood sugar that trigger inflammation, oxidative stress, and cartilage breakdown.

arachidonic acid: An omega-6 fat that is produced in the arachidonic acid pathway. A diet high in omega-6 fats leads to the formation of increased inflammation in the body.

C-reactive protein (CRP): A blood protein that becomes elevated in states of increased body inflammation.

erythrocyte sedimentation rate (ESR): A blood protein that is found to be elevated in states of increased inflammation in the body.

homocysteine: A chemical biomarker that, when elevated in the blood, indicates increased inflammation in the body. Elevated homocysteine can result from low B-complex vitamin intake and predisposes individuals to heart disease.

interleukin-1 (IL-1): An inflammatory cytokine that has an active role in cartilage breakdown.

interleukin-6 (IL-6): An inflammatory cytokine that has an active role in cartilage breakdown.

interleukin-1-beta (IL-1-beta): An inflammatory cytokine that is involved in cartilage destruction in joints with osteoarthritis.

leukotrienes: Inflammatory chemical compounds produced by cells. They are overproduced and are harmful when we consume excessive "bad" fats in our diet.

nitric oxide (NO): A chemical, produced in cartilage cells during states of increased oxidative stress, that stimulates cartilage breakdown.

omega-6 fats: A group of fats that lead to increased body inflammation when consumed excessively compared to healthy omega-3 fats. The classic American diet has increased omega-6 fats, which predisposes individuals to heart disease, high cholesterol, and increased inflammation.

TNF-alpha: A protein that increases inflammation in the body. It is an important inflammatory chemical messenger that causes cartilage breakdown in our joints.

VEGF: An inflammatory compound found in increased amounts in arthritic joints.

Glossary

abdominal obesity: Fat stored around the belly.

acetyl-L-carnitine (ALCAR): A naturally occurring chemical which can be used as a supplement to decrease oxidative stress or the "rusting" of our organs. When combined with another chemical, alpha lipoic acid, it decreases damage done to cells by free radicals and by the aging process.

ADAMTS (a disintegrin-like and metalloprotease with Thrombospondin motifs): A family of many enzymes which are cartilage degrading.

ADAMTS4: A cartilage-degrading enzyme that has an active role in osteoarthritis.

adenosine triphosphate (ATP): The chemical compound a cell uses for energy to power itself. Food is converted to energy in the body in the form of ATP, which is then used to carry out the chemical reactions in the body by providing the energy needed to build and maintain our organs.

adipocytokines: Fat-derived hormones that control fat and sugar metabolism in the body. Leptin and adiponectin are adipocytokines.

adiponectin: A hormone produced by fat cells whose levels are decreased in obesity and which plays a role in osteoarthritis.

adrenal glands: Organs that sit on top of the kidneys and regulate the "fight-or-flight" stress response in the body by producing the hormones cortisol and adrenaline.

advanced glycation endproducts (AGEs): Sugar-coated proteins formed by excess blood sugar that trigger inflammation, oxidative stress, and cartilage breakdown.

aggrecan: A major protein component of our three-dimensional cartilage framework.

aggrecanases: Enzymes found in cartilage that degrade cartilage by breaking down the protein aggrecan.

alpha lipoic acid (ALA): A chemical compound found naturally in vegetables such as spinach and broccoli. It can also be taken as a supplement, and it is an effective antioxidant that decreases the accumulation of damaging free radicals in cells.

anthocyanidins: A class of pigments that give plants their color, and are powerful antioxidants.

antioxidants: Substances that prevent the reaction of chemicals in cells with oxygen free radicals. This reaction causes cells to become oxidized and rancid. Antioxidants prevent the formation of "rust" in cells and help to fight oxidative stress.

arachidonic acid pathway: A set of chemical reactions in our cells that convert fats from our diet into chemical messengers called prostaglandins, which affect the inflammatory status of our bodies.

arteries: Blood vessels that carry oxygen-rich blood from the heart to rest of the body.

articular cartilage: The cartilage in our joints that cushions the joint and allows the joint to glide smoothly.

atherosclerosis: A condition caused by increased clotting and increased inflammation on blood vessel walls, leading to the buildup of sludge that blocks blood flow. It is also known as "hardening of the arteries."

automated DNA sequencers: The process of determining the order of nucleotides (G, C, A, T) on a DNA segment. The fragments of DNA are labeled using fluorescent dyes and a laser beam is passed over them. The color of each dye-labeled fragment is then determined with the use of a computer. This automated approach increases the speed by which DNA is analyzed.

avascular necrosis (AVN): A loss of blood supply to the bone that causes the bone to die.

avocado/soybean unsaponifiables (ASU): This compound is obtained from chemical processing of avocado and soybean oils, and it has powerful anti-inflammatory effects in the treatment of osteoarthritis.

beta-carotene: A compound that forms vitamin A. Carotenes give carrots their orange color.

bioflavonoids: Natural colorful pigments found in fruits and vegetables. They are powerful antioxidants and have anti-inflammatory properties.

biologic potentiality: This refers to the fact that our genetic makeup is influenced by the environment and nutrition. Our genetic predispositions are not set in stone.

biomarkers: Chemical compounds whose measurement in blood or organs is used to diagnose certain diseases.

biphosphonates: Drugs that prevent the loss of bone and are often used to treat osteoporosis.

body inflammation: An unhealthy chemical state in the body, of which one major cause is a diet containing high levels of sugars, empty-calorie carbohydrates, and unhealthy trans fats and saturated fats.

body mass index (BMI): A numeric guide used to classify our weight as normal, overweight, obese, or extremely obese. The numerial ranges are: 19–24, normal; 25–29, overweight; 30–39, obese; and 40–54, extremely obese.

bone mineral density (BMD): A measurement of the bone thickness, or mass, of our skeleton. A low BMD predisposes to easier breaking of bones and is seen in osteoporosis.

bromelain: A protein-breaking enzyme found in pineapples, which is an anti-inflammatory agent.

calcium ascorbate: A form of calcium supplement that also contains vitamin C.

cartilage: The cushion in our joints that is made up of cartilage cells and a three-dimensional collagen framework. It allows the smooth gliding of two bone surfaces past each other in order to move the skeleton.

cartilage cells: Cells that produce the cartilage that cushions our joints.

cartilage oligomeric matrix protein (COMP): A breakdown fragment of the cartilage matrix that is indicative of cartilage destruction.

catalase: An important detoxification enzyme that is responsible for eliminating toxic substances from the body.

cell membrane: A barrier which surrounds a cell and separates it from the outside environment. It receives chemical signals from other cells and transmits them to the DNA in the nucleus.

cells: The basic units of life that make up the organs in our body.

cetyl myristoleate (CMO): A chemical compound that decreases inflammation in osteoarthritis by blocking the COX and LOX enzymes in the arachidonic acid pathway.

chemical intermediates: These are often harmful chemicals produced in the detoxification process which need to be eliminated by the body by being converted to nontoxic compounds.

chondroitin: A nutraceutical that is beneficial in the treatment of osteoarthritis. It is normally found in cartilage and gives it a lot of its compressive strength. It makes up the aggrecan, which is a major component of cartilage.

chromium picolinate: A chemical substance that can be taken in supplement form and promotes the proper functioning of the hormone insulin in regulating our blood sugar.

coenzyme Q10: A chemical compound that helps mitochondria convert the food we eat into energy. It can be taken in supplement form and it has antioxidant properties, protecting cells from damaging free radicals.

collagen: The structural backbone of cartilage that becomes fragmented when cartilage is damaged in osteoarthritis.

collagen synthesis: Cartilage cells synthesize the three-dimensional structural protein which makes up the bulk of the cartilage.

cortisol: A hormone produced by the adrenal glands that is involved in regulating the "stress response" in the body. The stress response occurs when we face a certain danger, and it results in increased blood pressure and heart rate. Chronic stress produces chronically elevated cortisol and has damaging effects on the body.

COX-2: An important inflammation-producing enzyme in the arachidonic acid pathway. It produces inflammatory or "bad" prostaglandins that lead to pain. The nonsteroidal anti-inflammatory Vioxx, which was pulled off the market, works by blocking the COX-2 enzyme.

C-reactive protein (CRP): A blood protein that becomes elevated in states of increased body inflammation.

curcumin: Most commonly found in turmeric, the Indian spice used to make curry. It is a powerful antioxidant, anti-inflammatory, and blocks the production of cartilage degrading matrix metalloproteinase enzymes.

cytokines: Chemical messengers that transmit signals to our cells. IL-1 and TNF-alpha are bad cytokines that increase inflammation in our bodies. There are good and bad cytokines, and while the bad cytokines increase inflammation, the good cytokines help to decrease inflammation.

degrading substances: Chemical substances in the joints that break down cartilage.

detoxification enzyme systems: Systems in cells that clean up toxic buildup. When our diets are unhealthy, these enzymes start to malfunction, allowing free radicals to accumulate and cause damage.

DHA: The beneficial omega-3 fat found in fish oils from coldwater fish such as salmon and sardines.

diastolic blood pressure: The lower number in the blood pressure reading. In the case of a blood pressure of 130/80, 80 represents the pressure in our blood vessels in the resting phase of the heart when it is not pumping blood.

disease-modifying benefits: The ability of a nutraceutical to reverse or to stop the progression of the osteoarthritic damage in cartilage.

DNA: The blueprint of all the instructions needed to carry out the functions of the living organism. It is made up of long chains of chemical compounds called nucleotides, which code for specific information depending on the function of a given cell. These chains are intertwined into a helical configuration, which is why DNA is sometimes referred as a double helix.

double-blind scientific research: Research performed when neither the participants nor the researchers know who belongs in the control versus the experimental group. This is the most objective and unbiased way of doing scientific research that produces valid, reliable conclusions.

electron microscopy: An electron microscope is a specialized microscope that uses electrons to visualize very small objects such as individual cells, DNA segments, and mitochondria. It can magnify specimens up to 1–2 million times.

electrophoresis: A research method in which particles being studied, such as proteins, are separated. An electric current is used to disperse them in water, where they can be isolated and identified.

endocrine organs: The organs that produce compounds called hormones. Hormones regulate the body's chemical balance, or homeostasis.

enzymes: Proteins that carry out the multiple chemical reactions inside a cell.

EPA: The beneficial omega-3 fat found in fish oils from coldwater fish such as salmon and sardines.

epigenetic modification: Chemical changes that occur in our DNA which allow certain genes to be turned on and off. Nutrients have powerful effects on our genes by being able to chemically change portions of our DNA in this manner.

erythrocyte sedimentation rate (ESR): A blood protein that is found to be elevated in states of increased inflammation in the body.

essential amino acid: Amino acids are the building blocks of protein, and *essential* refers to certain amino acids that the body cannot manufacture and must be obtained from the food we eat.

evidence-based medicine: Medical treatments that have been scientifically proven to be effective and to be the best treatment for a particular condition.

fibronectin fragments: Fragments of cartilage which have powerful action in triggering further cartilage breakdown and in increasing the level of inflammation in joints.

flavonoids: Chemical substances in vegetables that give them their colorful appearance and are powerful antioxidants.

FN-f receptors: Receptors on cartilage cells that respond to cartilage breakdown fragments, known as fibronectin fragments, to trigger further activation of cartilage breakdown enzymes. This continues the vicious cycle of osteoarthritic cartilage breakdown.

folate (folic acid): Part of the B-vitamin-complex family that is found in fruits and vegetables. Adequate levels in the body are important in preventing the accumulation of the inflammatory compound homocysteine.

free radicals: Highly reactive compounds that steal electrons from other compounds and damage cells. They steal electrons because they have unpaired electrons, which leads them to take an electron from another compound in order to become balanced. In the process, the compounds in cells whose electron is stolen are damaged, leading to disease states.

G82S: A small change in the gene that produces the RAGE receptor. People with this SNP variation have a RAGE receptor that is more aggressive in triggering joint cartilage destruction.

gene chips: The technology of putting many microscopic DNA pieces on a solid surface through chemically attaching them to the surface of glass or silicon. These DNA segments are then used as probes, since they can identify similar DNA segments when exposed to them during genetic testing.

gene expression: The turning on of genes that allows them to produce their encoded proteins.

genes: Small segments of a DNA strand that contain the information to code for a specific protein. Every chemical compound in the cell is coded for by a specific gene.

glucosamine: A nutraceutical beneficial in the treatment of osteoarthritis. It is isolated from shellfish, and it is used to form glycosaminoglycans, which are a major component of cartilage.

GLUT-4 transport system: A chemical in the cell membrane of cells that picks up sugar from the blood and transports it inside the cell so it can be used as energy.

glutathione: A chemical compound that assists the enzyme glutathione peroxidase to perform detoxification functions in cells.

glutathione peroxidase: An important detoxification enzyme that is responsible for eliminating toxic substances from the body.

glycated collagen: "Sugar-coated" collagen, which is stiffer and more brittle, and thus breaks down more easily under stress than normal collagen. Glycated collagen accumulates in states of chronically elevated blood sugar levels.

green tea catechins: Chemical substances found in green tea that are antioxidants.

growth factors: A class of chemical compounds that regulate and maintain proper functioning of cells and body organs by acting as chemical messengers.

high-density lipoprotein (HDL): The type of cholesterol in the blood that is healthy. Elevated HDL levels help prevent heart disease.

high-glycemic-index carbohydrates: Foods that increase the blood sugar level very quickly. They are unhealthy because they lead to weight gain and elevated blood sugar, and predispose individuals to developing diabetes.

high-glycemic-load diets: Diets that contain high levels of sugar and other unhealthy carbohydrates. These foods, when consumed regularly, cause chronically elevated blood sugar and insulin levels, which predispose individuals to diabetes.

high-resolution nuclear magnetic resonance imaging: A specialized test that uses a magnetic field to measure the amounts of different chemicals present in the body's organs.

high-speed gene sequencing: Gene sequencing involves determining the order of nucleotides (G, C, A, T) on a segment of DNA. DNA fragments are tested by first labeling them with radioactivity or a fluorescent dye, and then analyzing their nucleotide content using a computer. In this manner, large amounts of DNA segments can be analyzed and decoded simultaneously.

high-throughput genotyping: The process of using computers to analyze multiple segments of DNA in order to create DNA libraries of every nucleotide in the sequence of DNA. The number of nucleotides in the whole human DNA is in the billions.

homeostasis: A state of optimum chemical balance in the body.

homocysteine: A chemical biomarker that, when elevated in the blood, indicates increased inflammation in the body. Elevated homocysteine can result from low B-complex vitamin intake and predisposes individuals to heart disease.

hormonal imbalance: When hormone levels in the body are not at appropriate levels relative to one another. Hormonal imbalance leads to disease.

hormones: Protein compounds produced in the body that regulate the many vital functions of living. They do this by acting as chemical transmitters that allow cells in the body to communicate with one another.

human genome: All the genes—about 25,000 to 30,000—that make up our DNA. It is the complete set of information in the human DNA.

hydrogen: The most common chemical element in nature. In osteoarthritis, damage is caused when unstable hydrogen-containing free radicals are produced.

hydrogenation: A chemical processing of fats used by the food industry in which hydrogen is added to oils to chemically modify them and make them hard. These are called trans fats and have increased shelf life.

hydrogen peroxide (H_2O_2): A common oxidizing agent found in cartilage cells that acts similarly to the bleach we use to wash clothes. The hydrogen peroxide in bleach clears the stains from clothes through an oxidation process; by removing hydrogen from other compounds, hydrogen peroxide damages them by causing them to become oxidized.

hypothalamus: A specialized part of the brain which contains a number of regulatory centers that control functions in the body not under conscious control, such as breathing, body temperature, and intestinal function.

IL-1 receptor antagonist (IL-1Ra): A chemical that blocks the effects of the inflammatory cytokine IL-1 and thus protects against cartilage breakdown.

inflammation: A set of chemical reactions in the body used by the body to fight foreign invaders and to heal injuries. When these inflammatory processes are chronically activated, they can lead to organ damage and the development of diseases.

inflammatory cytokines: Unhealthy chemical messengers that increase inflammation and cartilage breakdown in osteoarthritis.

inflammatory prostaglandins: Chemical messengers overproduced in the arachidonic acid pathway when we consume an excessive amount of unhealthy fats.

iNOS: The enzyme responsible for producing nitric oxide (NO), which causes oxidative damage in cartilage.

insulin: An important hormone whose main function in the body is to regulate blood sugar levels.

insulin growth factor-1 (IGF-1): A small chemical messenger protein needed to properly maintain healthy cartilage in our joints. Fifty percent of IGF-1 is lost between early adulthood and old age. This is detrimental to the proper maintenance of our organs such as cartilage.

insulin resistance: A state of dysfunction in which our cells cannot respond to insulin and are thus unable to absorb sugar from the bloodstream. This increased blood sugar (hyperglycemia) results in the formation of toxic advanced glycation endproducts, which damage many organs, including joint cartilage.

interleukin-1 (IL-1): An inflammatory cytokine that has an active role in cartilage breakdown.

interleukin-6 (IL-6): An inflammatory cytokine that has an active role in cartilage breakdown.

IRS-1: The insulin receptor found in the membrane of cells, which combines with the circulating hormone insulin and triggers cells to pick up sugar from the blood.

leptin: A fat-derived hormone that regulates the amount of fat in the body, controls hunger, and affects our inflammatory state. It is increased in osteoarthritis.

leptin receptor: A chemical compound located on the cartilage cell membrane that recognizes and binds leptin. This interaction signals the increased production of cartilage-degrading compounds.

leptin resistance: The increased production of leptin by inflamed fat cells in states of obesity and metabolic syndrome results in the inability of cells to appropriately respond to its messages. This state, in which cells are "deaf" to the messages of leptin, is unhealthy.

leukotrienes: Inflammatory chemical compounds produced by cells. They are overproduced and are harmful when we consume excessive "bad" fats in our diet.

leukotriene LTB4: A leukotriene that is involved in generating increased oxidative stress, through the increased production of free radicals in our joints.

low-density lipoprotein (LDL): An unhealthy type of cholesterol in the blood that, when elevated, predisposes individuals to heart disease.

LOX enzyme: An enzyme present in the arachidonic acid pathway of inflammation, it produces the inflammatory compounds known as leukotrienes.

lutein: A naturally occurring compound found in green leafy vegetables such as spinach.

lycopene: An antioxidant compound found in tomatoes.

MAPK: A chemical intermediate in cells that transmits inflammatory messages from hormones and "bad" prostaglandins to the DNA in our nuclei.

mass spectrometry: An experimental technique used to measure the concentration of chemicals in a solution. It is used to sequence DNA fragments and separate them based on size. This allows one to figure out the sequence of the nucleotides (G, C, A, T) that make up the DNA.

matrix metalloproteinases (MMPs): Cartilage-degrading enzymes whose production is increased by osteoarthritic cartilage cells and which are responsible for the destruction of cartilage.

Mediterranean diet: A diet high in healthy omega-3 fats, olive oil, nuts, vegetables, fruits, and red wine. Its benefits lie in the fact that it is high in "good" fats and also fruits and vegetables.

meta-analysis: The statistical analysis of combining the results of several studies in order to increase the statistical power and allow more accurate data interpretation.

metabolic acidosis: High levels of acidity in the body. This state is toxic to cells, causing them to malfunction.

metabolic syndrome: An unhealthy group of body parameters that include increased waist size, increased blood pressure, increased cholesterol and triglycerides, increased levels of blood sugar, and decreased good fat HDL. These predispose individuals to the development of inflammatory and degenerative diseases.

metabolic theory of osteoarthritis: The postulation that unhealthy diet, obesity, hormonal imbalance, and increased inflammation in the body lead to cartilage damage.

metabolism: The sum total of all chemical reactions that occur in the body and that sustain life.

metabolomics: The study of how nutrients in our diet affect chemical changes in the body. The chemical effects of diet are studied using high-resolution nuclear magnetic resonance imaging.

methionine: An amino acid that produces SAMe, an important agent in detoxification. It is obtained from foods such as fish, seeds, and Brazil nuts.

methylation: An important class of chemical reactions in the body that are involved in detoxification and gene expression. Methylation chemical reactions involving the DNA alter gene function by adding a methyl group (which is a carbon and hydrogen compound) on a portion of the DNA. Methylation is an important way in which diet and the environment affect our genes.

methylenetetrahydrofolate reductase (MTHFR): An important enzyme that eliminates the toxic chemical homocysteine from accumulating in our bodies. B-complex vitamins are helpers of this enzyme.

methylsulfonylmethane (MSM): A chemical compound that is beneficial in the treatment of osteoarthritis.

mitochondria: Energy-producing factories in cells that generate increased oxidative stress when they are not functioning well.

mitochondrial electron transport chain: The set of chemical reactions occurring in the mitochondria (the energy producing factories of our cells), which generates energy for the cell.

MMP-13: An enzyme produced by cartilage cells that breaks down cartilage.

N-acetylcysteine (NAC): An important antioxidant chemical that reduces the production of inflammatory compounds produced in the arachidonic acid pathway. It helps reduce inflammation in the body.

NADPH oxidase: An enzyme found in cartilage cells responsible for increasing oxidative stress by producing damaging free radicals.

NFkB: A chemical intermediate in cells that transmits inflammatory messages from "bad" prostaglandins to the DNA in our nuclei.

niacinamide: A form of vitamin B_3 that has anti-inflammatory properties. Research has shown that it is beneficial in treating osteoarthritis.

nitric oxide (NO): A chemical, produced in cartilage cells during states of increased oxidative stress, that stimulates cartilage breakdown.

nucleotide base pairs: A sugar-containing chemical compound linked together to form the double-stranded DNA structure.

nucleus: This is the storage warehouse of the genetic information of a cell, the DNA. It is the cell's command center.

nutraceuticals: Nutritional substances that are beneficial in treating and preventing disease.

nutrigenetics: The study of how gene variations affect the response of individuals to different nutrients and diets. It can be used to determine if a person's genetic makeup predisposes him or her to the development of disease.

nutrigenomics: The study of the effect of nutrition on our DNA. It studies how nutrients can turn certain genes on and off.

nutritional treatments: Nutraceuticals used to treat diseases such as osteoarthritis.

obesity: Increased body weight, which predisposes individuals to the development of degenerative and inflammatory diseases.

omega-3 fats: Healthful fats that decrease inflammation in the body when included in adequate amounts in our diet. They are also helpful in decreasing osteoarthritic cartilage breakdown and have beneficial effects on heart disease, diabetes, and elevated cholesterol.

omega-6 fats: A group of fats that lead to increased body inflammation when consumed excessively compared to healthy omega-3 fats. The classic American diet has increased omega-6 fats, which predisposes individuals to heart disease, high cholesterol, and increased inflammation.

oncostatin M: An inflammatory substance found in cartilage that causes cartilage damage by increasing the production of cartilage-degrading enzymes.

OPG/RANKL system: A set of coordinated chemical reactions found in bone whose job is to maintain the health and integrity of bone, by regulating the density (strength) of bone.

osteoblasts: Cells in bone that are responsible for manufacturing the hard framework of bone and in replacing aging bone.

osteoclasts: Cells in the bone that break down bone. They are involved in normal maintenance by replacing old with new bone.

osteoporosis: The most common bone disease which lowers the density (strength) of bone, and is seen most commonly in post-menopausal women as a result of loss of estrogen.

oxidation: This occurs when a chemical compound loses hydrogen ions in a chemical reaction with oxygen free radicals. By losing a hydrogen atom it also loses an electron, which damages the chemical compound.

oxidative stress: A "rusting" process in which oxygen free radicals cause tissue damage in cells by stealing electrons from other compounds, causing them to become oxidized. Oxidative stress plays an important role in the cartilage breakdown seen in osteoarthritis.

oxidizing agents: Chemical substances that give oxygen to another compound or steal hydrogen and electrons from that compound. Common oxidizing agents are oxygen and hydrogen peroxide. Important oxidizing agents in our joints are oxygen free radicals.

oxygen free radicals: Free radicals that contain oxygen. They are unstable compounds that steal electrons from other compounds, thus damaging the chemical machinery of the cell.

oxygen radical absorbent capacity (ORAC): A measure of a food's ability to neutralize damaging free radicals in our cells when eaten. Blueberries, cinnamon, and green tea have high ORAC values, and are powerful antioxidants that promote good health.

paradigm: The current way of thinking within the scientific community, which includes beliefs, biases, and the basic principles scientists use to explain phenomena. Paradigms can change as more and more new discoveries are made.

pentosan polysulfate (PPS): A semisynthetic glucosaminoglycan that has been shown to have cartilage-protective and blood-thinning properties.

pentosidine: An advanced glycation endproduct (AGE) that has been shown to accumulate in joint cartilage in osteoarthritis.

peroxisome proliferator-activated receptors (PPAR receptors): Receptors in cells that bind to chemicals, such as hormones and cytokines, and act to oppose the actions of inflammatory IL-1 and RAGE signals.

pharmacogenomics: An emerging field that studies how people's individual genetic makeup allows them to process and eliminate drugs they are taking.

polypharmancy: The multiple drugs taken, especially by the elderly, which can interact with one another and cause side effects.

polyphenols: Chemical compounds found in plants that are powerful antioxidants.

polyunsatured fats: Fats, including omega-3 and omega-6 fats, found in meats, grains, fish oil, and soy. The key to polyunsaturated fats is to eat the right balance of omega-3 to omega-6 fats in order to be healthy. Eating too many omega-6 fats compared to omega-3s predisposes individuals to increased inflammation and disease in the body.

positive carryover effect: Beneficial effect of nutraceuticals, such as glucosamine and chondroitin, which is their ability to help joints even after they have ceased to be consumed for a period of months.

PPAR-alpha: A specialized cell receptor found on the cell membrane that conveys information to the DNA. When it is activated by "good" omega-3 fats, it acts to lower inflammation in the body.

PPAR-delta: A receptor found on the surface of cells that interacts with the hormone estrogen to dampen the inflammatory response.

PPAR-gamma: A specialized chemical that, when stimulated in cartilage cells, opposes the action of inflammatory cytokines such as IL-1.

pre-diabetes: A state of insulin resistance in which blood sugar levels are chronically elevated in the body.

prostaglandins: Chemical compounds that are important messengers in cellular communication. Inflammatory prostaglandins are involved in the degrading cycle of osteoarthritic cartilage breakdown.

proteases: Proteins produced by cartilage cells that break down and remove aging cartilage and replace it with new cartilage.

proteins: The building blocks of all structures in the body. Proteins comprise one of the three classes of important compounds; the other two are fats and carbohydrates.

proteoglycans: Subunits that make up the three-dimensional cartilage matrix by combining with collagen and water.

proteomics: The study of the interactions of proteins in order to discover their function and relation to other proteins in cells.

RAGE receptors: Found on the surface of cartilage cells, these initiate cartilage breakdown when they bind advanced glycation end-products (AGEs).

retinoids: Derivatives of vitamin A that block the genes that produce cartilage breakdown enzymes (matrix metalloproteinases).

rhinoviruses: The most common viruses to infect humans, they are the cause of the "common cold."

rust: A chemical substance made of iron oxide. This rusting process is an oxidation reaction found in cells such as cartilage cells, and it leads to destruction by a process known as oxidative stress.

salicylates: Painkilling drugs of which acetylsalicylic acid or aspirin is the best known.

saturated fats: These are fats made of triglycerides that are found in foods such as meats, butter, eggs, milk, and cheese. Diets high in saturated fats increase blood cholesterol and are linked to the development of clogging of the arteries and heart disease.

single nucleotide polymorphisms (SNPs): Small changes in the sequence of a gene that lead that gene to code for a protein with altered function. It is SNPs in key genes that predispose people to develop certain diseases.

sirtuins: Life-extending genes that are activated by trans-resveratrol (an antioxidant compound found in red wine) when given to mice.

SOCS-3: A chemical compound that blocks the hormone leptin's ability to communicate with cells.

soy isoflavones: Antioxidants found in soy products, which fight osteoarthritis.

steroids: Powerful inhibitors of the degrading enzymes in cartilage, the matrix metalloproteinases. They have powerful actions in improving arthritis pain and inflammation, but with many side effects.

subchondral bone: The bone on which articular cartilage rests in our joints.

sugar-coated proteins: Excess amounts of circulating blood sugar can coat important proteins, such as those in cartilage, causing weakening and breakdown of joints.

superoxide dismutase: An important detoxification enzyme that is responsible for eliminating toxic substances from the body. It prevents the accumulation of free radicals and thus decreases oxidative stress in cartilage cells.

synergism: The phenomenon in which the benefits of combining nutraceuticals in treating osteoarthritis exceed the benefits of consuming each one alone.

synovial fluid: Fluid found in our joints that bathes cartilage and delivers nutrients to cartilage cells. It is the lubricating fluid found in joints.

systolic blood pressure: The upper number in the blood pressure reading. In the case of a blood pressure of 130/80, the 130 represents the pressure exerted by the heart in pumping blood through the body.

thromboxanes: Inflammatory chemical compounds produced by cells in the arachidonic acid pathway.

TNF-alpha: A protein that increases inflammation in the body. It is an important inflammatory chemical messenger that causes cartilage breakdown in our joints.

total joint replacement: A surgical procedure used in severe cases of osteoarthritis to remove all diseased cartilage and replace it with metal and plastic components.

trans-resveratrol: A powerful antioxidant found in red wine. Large doses injected in joints of arthritic mice decrease cartilage destruction in osteoarthritis.

triglycerides: These are fats found in our blood; fat from foods is stored in cells to be later used as energy. When triglyerides in blood are elevated, they predispose individuals to metabolic syndrome.

triterpenoids: Plant compounds that inhibit the genes that produce the cartilage-degrading matrix metalloproteinases. They also block the inflammation-producing COX and LOX enzymes in the arachidonic acid pathway.

two-dimensional electrophoresis: Proteins are placed on a specialized gel surface, and an electric current is applied in order to separate them from each other. Analysis can thus be made as to which proteins are present and at which concentration.

type 2 diabetes: A disease caused when the pancreas does not produce enough insulin, the hormone needed to properly process the sugar we consume. This leads to increased blood sugar, which in turn damages organs in our body.

VEGF: An inflammatory compound found in increased amounts in arthritic joints.

veins: Blood vessels that return blood from the organs to the heart.

xanthines: Chemicals found in teas and coffee that stimulate the brain and relax the blood vessels.

Notes

INTRODUCTION: OSTEOARTHRITIS: WHAT IT IS AND ITS IMPACT ON SOCIETY

1. L. S. Simon, "Update in Osteoarthritis," *Med GenMed e Journal* (November 26, 2003).

2. L. Meszaros, "Orthopedic Update," *Greater Sacramento M.D. News* (November/December 2006): 8.

3. E. S. Ford, W. H. Giles, and W. H. Dietz, "Prevalence of the Metabolic Syndrome among U.S. Adults: Findings from the Third National Health and Nutrtion Examination Survey," *Journal of the American Medical Association* 287, no. 3 (2002): 356–59.

4. Ibid.

5. G. W. Duff, "Evidence for Genetic Variation as a Factor in Maintaining Health," *American Journal of Clinical Nutrition* 83, supp. (2006): 431S–435S.

6. T. T. Perls, "The Different Paths to 100," *American Journal of Clinical Nutrition* 83, supp. (2006): 484S–487S.

7. J. A. Buckwalter, C. Saltzman, and T. Brown, "The Impact of Osteoarthritis: Implications for Research," *Clinical Orthopaedics and Related Research* 427, supp. (2004): S6–S15.

8. W. Cai et al., "High Levels of Dietary Advanced Glycation End Products Transform Low-Density Lipoprotein into a Potent Redox-Sensitive Mitogen-Activated Protein Kinase Stimulant in Diabetic Patients," *Circulation* 110 (2004): 285–91.

9. D. L. Cecil et al., "Inflammation-Induced Chondrocyte Hypertrophy Is Driven by Receptor for Advanced Glycation End Products," *Journal of Immunology* 175, no. 12 (2005): 8296–8302.

CHAPTER 1: CARTILAGE AND ITS ROLE IN OSTEOARTHRITIS

1. P. E. DiCesare et al., "Matrix-Matrix Interaction of Cartilage Oligomeric Matrix Protein and Fibronectin," *Matrix Biology* 21, no. 5 (2002): 461–70.

2. M. B. Goldring and F. Berenbaum, "The Regulation of Chondrocyte Function by Pro-Inflammatory Mediators," *Clinical Orthopaedics and Related Research* 427, supp. (2004): S37–S46.

3. B. N. Ames, "Delaying the Mitochondrial Decay of Aging," *Annals of the New York Academy of Sciences* 1019 (2004): 406–11.

4. M. Fenech, "Micronutrients and Genomic Stability: A New Paradigm for Recommended Dietary Allowances (RDAs)," *Food and Chemical Toxicology* 40, no. 8 (2002): 1113–17.

5. Ibid.

6. J. C. Fernandes, J. Martel-Pelletier, and J.-P. Pelletier, "The Role of Cytokines in Osteoarthritis Pathophysiology," *Biorheology* 39, no. 1–2 (2002): 237–46.

7. Fenech, "Micronutrients and Genomic Stabiligy."

8. L. J. Sandell and T. Aigner, "Articular Cartilage and Changes in Arthritis. An Introduction: Cell Biology of Osteoarthritis," *Arthritis Research* 3 (2001): 107–13.

9. Ibid.

10. J.-P. Pelletier et al., "The Protective Effect of Licofelone on Experimental Osteoarthritis Is Correlated with the Downregulation of Gene Expression and Protein Synthesis of Several Major Catabolic Factors: MMP-13, Cathepsin K and Aggrecanases," *Arthritis Research and Therapy* 7, no. 5 (2005): R1091–R1102.

11. R. F. Loeser, "Aging Cartilage and Osteoarthritis—What's the Link?" *Science of Aging Knowledge Environment* 2004, no. 29 (2004): pe31.

12. C. B. Knudson and W. Knudson, "Hyaluronan and CD44: Modulators of Chondrocyte Metabolism," *Clinical Orthopaedics and Related Research* 427, supp. (2004): S152–S162; S. Ohno et al., "Hyaluronan Oligosaccharides Induce Matrix Metalloproteinase 13 via Transcriptional Activation of NFkappaB and p38 MAP Kinase in Articular Chondrocytes," *Journal of Biological Chemistry* 281, no. 26 (2006): 17952–60.

13. S. Rashad et al., "Effect of Non-steroidal Anti-inflammatory Drugs on the Course of Osteoarthritis," *Lancet* 2, no. 8662 (1989): 519–22.

14. K. D. Brandt, "Effects of Non-steroidal Anti-inflammatory Drugs on Chondrocyte Metabolism In Vitro and In Vivo," *American Journal of the Medical Sciences* 83, no. 5A (1987): 29–34.

15. P. Ghosh, "Evaluation of Disease Progression During Non-steroidal Anti-inflammatory Drug Treatment: Experimental Models," *Osteoarthritis and Cartilage* 7, no. 3 (1999): 340–42; J. T. Dingle, "Cartilage Maintenance in Osteoarthritis: Interaction of Cytokines, NSAID and Prostaglandins in Articular Cartilage Damage and Repair," *Journal of Rheumatology* 28, supp. (1991): 30–37.

16. M. Hasson, "NSAIDs and COX-2 Inhibitors Impede Tendon, Bone, and Cartilage Repair," *Orthopedics Today* (September 2006): 49–50.

CHAPTER 2: WHAT IS INSULIN RESISTANCE?

1. B. Sanda, "The Double Danger of High Fructose Corn Syrup," *Well-Being Journal* 16, no. 3 (2007): 15; P. Mohanty et al., "Glucose Challenge Stimulates Reactive Oxygen Species (ROS) Generation by Leukocytes," *Journal of Clinical Endocrinology and Metabolism* 85, no. 8 (2000): 2970–73.

2. H. Vlassara, "Advanced Glycation in Health and Disease: Role of the Modern Environment," *Annals of the New York Academy of Sciences* 1043 (2005): 452–60.

3. K. Esposito and D. Giugliano, "Diet and Inflammation: A Link to Metabolic and Cardiovascular Diseases," *European Heart Journal* 27 (2006): 15–20; K. F. Petersen and G. I. Shulman, "Etiology of Insulin Resistance," *American Journal of Medicine* 119, no. 5A (2006): 10S–16S.

4. S. Moschos, J. A. Mantozoros, and S. B. Christos, "The Emerging Clinical Significance of Leptin in Humans with Absolute and Relative Deficiency," *Current Opinion in Internal Medicine* 4, no. 6 (2005): 596–601.

5. W. Cai et al., "High Levels of Dietary Advanced Glycation End Products Transform Low-Density Lipoprotein into a Potent Redox-Sensitive Mitogen-Activated Protein Kinase Stimulant in Diabetic Patients," *Circulation* 110 (2004): 285–91.

6. A. G. Pittas, N. A. Joseph, and A. S. Greenberg, "Adipocytokines and Insulin Resistance," *Journal of Clinical Endocrinology and Metabolism* 89, no. 2 (2004): 447–52.

7. M. Otero et al., "Signalling Pathway Involved in Nitric Oxide Synthase type II Activation in Chondrocytes: Synergistic Effect of Leptin with Interleukin-1," *Arthritis Research and Therapy* 7 (2005): R581–R591.

8. M. M. Newkirk et al., "Advanced Glycation End Product (AGE)-Damaged IgG and IgM Autoantibodies to IgG-AGE in Patients with Early Synovitis," *Arthritis Research and Therapy* 5 (2003): R82–R90.

9. S. F. Yan et al., "Glycation, Inflammation, and RAGE: A Scaffold for the Macrovascular Complications of Diabetes and Beyond," *Circulation Research* 93, no. 12 (2003): 1159–69; P. Odetti et al., "Advanced Glycation End Products and Bone Loss During Aging," *Annals of the New York Academy of Sciences* 1043 (2005: 710–17; M. Brownlee, "Advanced Protein Glycosylation in Diabetes and Aging," *Annual Review of Medicine* 46 (1995): 223–34.

10. D. L. Cecil et al., "Inflammation-Induced Chondrocyte Hypertrophy Is Driven by Receptor for Advanced Glycation End Products," *Journal of Immunology* 175, no. 12 (2005): 8296–8302.

11. M. E. Obrenovich and U. M. Monnier, "Apoptotic Killing of Fibroblasts by Matrix-Bound Advanced Glycation End Products," *Science of Aging Knowledge Environment* 2005, no. 4 (2005): pe3.

12. Cecil et al., "Inflammation-Induced Chondrocyte Hypertrophy Is Driven by Receptor for Advanced Glycation End Products."

13. R. F. Loeser et al., "Articular Chondrocytes Express the Receptor for Advanced Glycation End Products: Potential Role in Osteoarthritis," *Arthritis and Rheumatism* 52, no. 8 (2005): 2376–85.

14. R. Ramasamy et al., "Advanced Glycation End Products and RAGE: A Common Thread in Aging, Diabetes, Neurodegeneration, and Inflammation," *Glycobiology* 15, no. 7 (2005): 16R–28R.

15. Z. Alikhani et al., "Advanced Glycation End Products Enhance Expression of Pro-apoptotic Genes and Stimulate Fibroblast Apoptosis through Cytoplasmic and Mitochondrial Pathways," *Journal of Biological Chemistry* 280, no. 13 (2005): 12087–95.

16. S. D. Phinney et al., "Abnormal Polyunsaturated Lipid Metabolism in the Obese Zucker Rat, with Partial Metabolic Correction by Gamma-Linolenic Acid Administration," *Metabolism* 42 (1993): 1127–40.

17. W. T. Cefalu et al., "Oral Chromium Picolinate Improves Carbohydrate and Lipid Metabolism and Enhances Skeletal Muscle GLUT-4 Translocation in Obese, Hyperinsulinemic (JCR-LA Corpulent) Rats," *Journal of Nutrition* 132 (2002): 1107–14.

18. T. You et al., "Abdominal Adipose Tissue Cytokine Gene Expression: Relationship to Obesity and Metabolic Risk Factors," *American Journal of Physiology Endocrinology and Metabolism* 288 (2005): E741–E747.

19. Pittas, Joseph, and Greenberg, "Adipocytokines and Insulin Resistance."

20. B. Lange-Sperandio et al., "RAGE Signaling in Cell Adhesion and Inflammation," *Current Pediatric Reviews* 3, no. 1 (2007): 1–9.

CHAPTER 3: WHAT IS OXIDATIVE STRESS?

1. W. Cai et al., "High Levels of Dietary Advanced Glycation End Products Transform Low-Density Lipoprotein into a Potent Redox-Sensitive Mitogen-Activated Protein Kinase Stimulant in Diabetic Patients," *Circulation* 110 (2004): 285–91; J. Uribarri et al., "Diet-Derived Advanced Glycation End Products Are Major Contributors to the Body's AGE Pool and Induce Inflammation in Healthy Subjects," *Annals of the New York Academy of Sciences* 1043 (2005): 461–66.

2. T. E. McAlindon, "Nutraceuticals: Do They Work and When Should We Use Them?" *Best Practice and Research Clinical Rheumatology* 20, no. 1 (2006): 99–115; K. B. Beckman and B. N. Ames, "The Free Radical Theory of Aging Matures," *Physiological Reviews* 78, no. 2 (1998): 547–81.

3. M. B. Goldring and F. Berenbaum, "The Regulation of Chondrocyte Function by Pro-inflammatory Mediators: Prostaglandins and Nitric Oxide," *Clinical Orthopaedics and Related Research* 427, supp. (2004): S37–S46; K. Sasaki et al., "Nitric Oxide Mediates Interleukin-1-Induced Gene Expression of Matrix Metalloproteinases and Basic Fibroblast Growth Factor in Cultured Rabbit Articular Chondrocytes," *Journal of Biochemistry* (*Tokyo*) 123 (1998): 431–39; R. Studer et al., "Nitric Oxide in Osteoarthritis," *Osteoarthritis and Cartilage* 7 (1999): 377–79; M. Oh M et al., "Concurrent Generation of Nitric Oxide and Superoxide Inhibits Proteoglycan Synthesis in Bovine Articular Chondrocytes: Involvement of Peroxynitrite," *Journal of Rheumatology* 25

(1998): 2169–74; M. R. van der Harst et al., "Nitrite and Nitrotyrosine Concentrations in Articular Cartilage, Subchondral Bone, and Trabecular Bone of Normal Juvenile, Normal Adult, and Osteoarthritic Adult Equine Metacarpophalangeal Joints," *Journal of Rheumatology* 33, no. 8 (2006): 1662–67.

4. P. Lane and S. S. Gross, "Cell Signaling by Nitric Oxide," *Seminars in Nephrology* 19, no. 3 (1999): 215–29.

5. A. Amin and S. Abramson, "The Role of Nitric Oxide in Articular Cartilage Breakdown in Osteoarthritis," *Current Opinion in Rheumatology* 10 (1998): 263–68.

6. K. Yudoh et al., "Potential Involvement of Oxidative Stress in Cartilage Senescence and Development of Osteoarthritis: Oxidative Stress Induces Chondrocyte Telomere Instability and Downregulation of Chondrocyte Function," *Arthritis Research and Therapy* 7 (2005): R380–R391.

7. C. B. Knudson and W. Knudson, "Hyaluronan and CD44: Modulators of Chondrocyte Metabolism," *Clinical Orthopaedics and Related Research* 427, supp. (2004): S152–S162.

8. J. A. Martin et al., "Chondrocyte Senescence, Joint Loading and Osteoarthritis," *Clinical Orthopaedics and Related Research* 427, supp. (2004): S96–S103; G. Kaiki et al., "Osteoarthrosis Induced by Intra-articular Hydrogen Peroxide Injection and Running Load," *Journal of Orthopaedic Research* 8, no. 5 (1990): 731–40.

9. Martin et al., "Chondrocyte Senescence."

10. M. C. Polidori, "Antioxidant Micronutrients in the Prevention of Age-Related Diseases," *Journal of Postgraduate Medicine* 49, no. 3 (2003): 229–35.

11. J. E. Upritchard et al., "Spread Supplemented with Moderate Doses of Vitamin E and Carotenoids Reduces Lipid Peroxidation in Healthy, Non-smoking Adults," *American Journal of Clinical Nutrition* 78 (2003): 985–92; I. Jialal, S. Devaraj, and S. K. Venugopal, "Oxidative Stress, Inflammation, and Diabetic Vasculopathies: The Role of Alpha-Tocopherol Therapy," *Free Radical Research* 36, no. 12 (2002): 1331–36.

12. K. Furomoto et al., "Age-Dependent Telomere Shortening Is Slowed Down by Enrichment of Intracellular Vitamin C via Suppression of Oxidative Stress," *Life Sciences* 63 (1998): 935–48.

13. S. Deakin et al., "Paraoxonase-1 Promoter Haplotypes and Serum Paraoxonase: A Predominant Role for Polymorphic Position-107, Implicating the Sp1 Transcription Factor," *Biochemical Journal* 372 (2003): 643–49.

14. K. S. Kornman, "Interleukin 1 Genetics, Inflammatory Mechanisms,

and Nutrigenic Opportunities to Modulate Diseases of Aging," *American Journal of Clinical Nutrition* 83, supp. (2006): 475S–483S.

15. P. J. Stover, "Influence of Human Genetic Variation on Nutritional Requirements," *American Journal of Clinical Nutrition* 83, supp. (2006): 436S–442S.

CHAPTER 4: EXCESS INFLAMMATION IS A SETUP FOR DISEASE IN THE JOINTS

1. J. Uribarri et al., "Diet-Derived Advanced Glycation End Products Are Major Contributors to the Body's AGE Pool and Induce Inflammation in Healthy Subjects," *Annals of the New York Academy of Sciences* 1043 (2005): 461–66; K. Esposito and D. Giugliano, "Diet and Inflammation: A Link to Metabolic and Cardiovascular Diseases," *European Heart Journal* 27, no. 1 (2006): 15–20.

2. M.-E. Pinche et al., "Relation of High-Sensitivity C-Reactive Protein, Interleukin-6. Tumor Necrosis Factor-Alpha, and Fibrinogen to Abdominal Adipose Tissue, Blood Pressure, and Cholesterol and Triglyceride Levels in Healthy Post-menopausal Women," *American Journal of Cardiology* 96, no. 1 (2005): 92–97; S. M. Grundy, "Obesity, Metabolic Syndrome, and Cardiovascular Disease," *Journal of Clinical Endocrinology and Metabolism* 89, no. 6 (2004): 2595–600.

3. P. A. Kern et al., "Adipose Tissue Tumor Necrosis Factor and Interleukin-6 Expression in Human Obesity and Insulin Resistance," *American Journal of Physiology* 280 (2001): E745–E751.

4. G. Davi et al., "Platelet Activation in Obese Women: Role of Inflammation and Oxidant Stress," *Journal of the American Medical Association* 288, no. 16 (2002): 2008–14; P. Ferroni et al., "Inflammation, Insulin Resistance, and Obesity," *Current Atherosclerosis Reports* 6 (2004): 424–31.

5. A. S. Greenberg and M. S. Obin, "Obesity and the Role of Adipose Tissue in Inflammation and Metabolism," *American Journal of Clinical Nutrition* 83, supp. (2006): 461S–465S.

6. A. P. Simopoulos, "The Mediterranean Diets: What Is so Special about the Diet of Greece? The Scientific Evidence," *Journal of Nutrition* 131 (2001): 3065S–3073S.

7. B. Watzl et al., "A 4-Week Intervention with High Intake Carotenoid-Rich Vegetables and Fruit Reduces Plasma C-Reactive Protein in Healthy Non-smoking Men," *American Journal of Clinical Nutrition* 82, no. 5 (2005): 1052–58.

CHAPTER 5: WHAT IS METABOLIC SYNDROME AND HOW IS IT RELATED TO OSTEOARTHRITIS?

1. P. Dandona et al., "Metabolic Syndrome: A Comprehensive Perspective Based on Interactions Between Obesity, Diabetes, and Inflammation," *Circulation* 111 (2005): 1448–54.

2. Expert Panel on Detection, Evaluation and Treatment of High Blood Cholesterol in Adults, "Executive Summary of the Third Report of the National Cholesterol Education Program (NCEP) Expert Panel on Detection, Evaluation, and Treatment of High Blood Cholesterol in Adults (Adult Treatment Panel III)," *Journal of the American Medical Association* 285 (2001): 2486–97.

3. E. S. Ford, W. H. Giles, and W. H. Dietz, "Prevalence of the Metabolic Syndrome among U.S. Adults: Findings from the Third National Health and Nutrition Examination Survey," *Journal of the American Medical Association* 287, no. 3 (2002): 356–59.

4. R. H. Knopp and P. Paramsothy, "Oxidized LDL and Abdominal Obesity: A Key to Understanding the Metabolic Syndrome," *American Journal of Clinical Nutrition* 83 (2006): 1–2.

5. L. W. Johnson and R. S. Weinstock, "The Metabolic Syndrome: Concepts and Controversy," *Mayo Clinic Proceedings* 81, no. 12 (2006): 1615–20.

6. M. Fenech, "Micronutrients and Genomic Stability: A New Paradigm for Recommended Dietary Allowances (RDAs)," *Food and Chemical Toxicology* 40, no. 8 (2002): 1113–17.

7. Ibid.

CHAPTER 6: OBESITY IS A BAD PLAYER IN THE DEGENERATION OF OUR JOINTS

1. World Health Organization, "WHO Global Database on BMI," *World Health Statistics*, 2007.

2. D. Starkey, "Medical Approach to Obesity Walks Line between Diet, Surgery," *Sacramento Business Journal*, December 1, 2006, 24.

3. G. Wheeler, "Chronic Conditions, Obesity. Main Factors behind Medical Spending Growth over Last 15 Years," *USA Today*, August 22, 2006.

4. Ibid.

5. G. Davi et al., "Platelet Activation in Obese Women: Role of Inflammation and Oxidant Stress," *Journal of the American Medical Association* 288, no. 16 (2002): 2008–14; T. You et al., "Abdominal Adipose Tissue Cytokine Gene Expression: Relationship to Obesity and Metabolic Risk Factors," *American Journal of Physiology Endocrinology and Metabolism* 288 (2005): E741–E747.

6. S. P. Weisberg et al., "Obesity Is Associated with Macrophage Accumulation in Adipose Tissue," *Journal of Clinical Investigation* 112 (2003): 1796–808; H. Xu et al., "Chronic Inflammation in Fat Plays a Crucial Role in the Development of Obesity-Related Insulin Resistance," *Journal of Clinical Investigation* 112 (2003): 1821–30.

7. A. M. Sharma, "The Obese Patient with Diabetes Mellitus: From Research Targets to Treatment Options," *American Journal of Medicine* 119, no. 5A (2006): 17S–23S; A. Schaffler et al., "Role of Adipose Tissue as an Inflammatory Organ in Human Diseases," *Endocrine Reviews* 27, no. 5 (2006): 449–67.

8. A. G. Pittas, N. A. Joseph, and A. S. Greenberg, "Adipocytokines and Insulin Resistance," *Journal of Clinical Endocrinology and Metabolism* 89, no. 2 (2004): 447–52.

9. Xu et al., "Chronic Inflammation"; P. Dandona, "Inflammation: The Link between Insulin Resistance, Obesity, and Diabetes," *Trends in Immunology* 25 (2004): 4–7. E. Lopez-Garcia et al., "Consumption of Trans Fatty Acids Is Related to Plasma Biomarkers of Inflammation and Endothelial Dysfunction," *Journal of Nutrition* 135 (2005): 562–66; D. Mozaffarian et al., "Trans-Fatty Acids and Systemic Inflammation in Heart Failure," *American Journal of Clinical Nutrition* 80 (2004): 1521–25.

CHAPTER 7: OXIDATIVE STRESS AND OSTEOARTHRITIS

1. U. Hoppe et al., "Coenzyme Q10, a Cutaneous Antioxidant and Energizer," *BioFactors* 9, no. 2–4 (1999): 371–78.

2. M. L. Tiku, R. Shah, and G. T. Allison, "Evidence Linking Chondrocyte Lipid Peroxidation to Cartilage Matrix Protein Degradation: Possible Role in Cartilage Aging and the Pathogenesis of Osteoarthritis," *Journal of Biological Chemistry* 275, no. 26 (2000): 20069–76; R. F. Loeser et al., "Detection of Nitrotyrosine in Aging and Osteoarthritic Cartilage: Correlation of Oxidative Damage with the Presence of Interleukin-1 Beta and with Chondrocyte Resistance to Insulin-Like Growth Factor-1," *Arthritis and Rheumatism* 46, no. 9 (2002): 2349–57.

3. Y. Henrotin et al., "Active Oxygen Species, Articular Inflammation, and Cartilage Damage," *EXS* 62 (1992): 308–22; Y. Henrotin et al., "Production of Active Oxygen Species by Isolated Human Chondrocytes," *British Journal of Rheumatology* 32, no. 7 (1993): 562–67.

4. B. Frel, "Reactive Oxygen Species and Antioxidant Vitamins: Mechanisms of Action," *American Journal of Medicine* 97, supp. 3A (1994): 5S–13S.

5. K. Yudoh et al., "Potential Involvement of Oxidative Stress in Cartilage Senescence and Development of Osteoarthritis: Oxidative Stress Induces Chondrocyte Telomere Instability and Downregulation of Chondrocyte Function," *Arthritis Research and Therapy* 7 (2005): R380–R391.

6. Tiku, Shah, and Allison, "Evidence Linking Chondrocyte Lipid Peroxidation to Cartilage Matrix Protein Degradation."

7. H. Xu et al., "Chronic Inflammation in Fat Plays a Crucial Role in the Development of Obesity-Related Insulin Resistance," *Journal of Clinical Investigation* 112 (2003): 1821–30; G. S. Hotamisligil, N. S. Shargill, and B. M. Spiegelman, "Adipose Expression of Tumor Necrosis Factor-Alpha: Direct Role in Obesity-Linked Insulin Resistance," *Science* 259 (1993): 87–91.

8. P. Dandona et al., "The Suppressive Effect of Dietary Restriction and Weight Loss in the Obese on the Generation of Reactive Oxygen Species by Leukocytes, Lipid Peroxidation, and Protein Carbonylation," *Journal of Clinical Endocrinology and Metabolism* 86, no. 1 (2001): 355–62.

9. G. Davi et al., "Platelet Activation in Obese Women: Role of Inflam-

mation and Oxidant Stress," *Journal of the American Medical Association* 288, no. 16 (2002): 2008–14.

10. P. Dandona et al., "Metabolic Syndrome: A Comprehensive Perspective Based on Interactions between Obesity, Diabetes, and Inflammation," *Circulation* 111 (2005): 1448–54.

CHAPTER 8: INFLAMMATION AND OSTEOARTHRITIS: A "FIVE-ALARM FIRE" IN OUR JOINTS

1. K. Esposito et al., "Inflammatory Cytokine Concentrations Are Acutely Increased by Hyperglycemia in Humans: Role of Oxidative Stress," *Circulation* 106 (2002): 2067.

2. H. Xu et al., "Chronic Inflammation in Fat Plays a Crucial Role in the Development of Obesity-Related Insulin Resistance," *Journal of Clinical Investigation* 112 (2003): 1821–30; M. E. Pinche et al., "Relation of High-Sensitivity C-Reactive Protein, Interleukin-6, Tumor Necrosis Factor-Alpha, and Fibrinogen to Abdominal Adipose Tissue, Blood Pressure, and Cholesterol and Triglyceride Levels in Healthy Post-menopausal Women," *American Journal of Cardiology* 96, no. 1 (2005): 92–97.

3. J. B. Catterall et al., "Synergistic Induction of Matrix Metalloproteinase-1 by Interleukin-1 Alpha and Oncostatin M in Human Chondrocytes Involves Signal Transducer and Activator of Transcription and Activator Protein-1 Transcription Factors via a Novel Mechanism," *Arthritis and Rheumatism* 44, no. 10 (2001): 2296–310; M. M. Temple et al., "Interleukin-1 Alpha Induction of Tensile Weakening Associated with Collagen Degradation in Bovine Articular Cartilage," *Arthritis and Rheumatism* 54, no. 10 (2006): 3267–76.

4. C. A. Dinarello, "Interleukin 1 and Interleukin 18 as Mediators of Inflammation and the Aging Process," *American Journal of Clinical Nutrition* 83, supp. (2006): 447S–455S.

5. K. S. Kornman, "Interleukin 1 Genetics, Inflammatory Mechanisms, and Nutrigenic Opportunities to Modulate Diseases of Aging," *American Journal of Clinical Nutrition* 83, supp. (2006): 475S–483S.

6. N. Fukui et al., "Stimulation of BMP-2 Expression by Pro-Inflammatory

Cytokines IL-1 and TNF-Alpha in Normal and Osteoarthritic Chondrocytes," *Journal of Bone and Joint Surgery (American)* 85 (2003): 59–66.

7. C. J. Malemud, N. Islam, and T. M. Haggi, "Pathophysiological Mechanisms in Osteoarthritis Lead to Novel Therapeutic Strategies," *Cells Tissues Organs* 174, no. 12 (2003): 34–48; C. Merrihew et al., "Modulation of Endogenous Osteogenic Protein-1 (OP-1) by Interleukin-1 in Adult Human Articular Cartilage," *Journal of Bone and Joint Surgery (American)* 85 (2003): 67–74.

8. C. B. Forsyth et al., "Increased Matrix Metalloproteinase-13 Production with Aging by Human Articular Chondrocytes in Response to Catabolic Stimuli," *Journals of Gerontology Series A: Biological Sciences and Medical Sciences* 60, no. 9 (2005): 1118–24.

9. H.-J. Im et al., "Inhibitory Effects of Insulin-Like Growth Factor-1 and Osteogenic Protein-1 on Fibronectin Fragment-and Interleukin-1 beta-Stimulated Matrix Metalloproteinase-13 Expression in Human Chondrocytes," *Journal of Biological Chemistry* 278, no. 28 (2003): 25386–94; T. Matsumoto et al., "Identification and Characterization of Insulin-Like Growth Factors (IGFs), IGF-Binding Proteins (IGFBPs) and IGFBP Proteases in Human Synovial Fluid," *Journal of Clinical Endocrinology and Metabolism* 81 (1996): 150–55; J. A. Martin et al., "Co-localization of Insulin-Like Growth Factor Binding Protein 3 and Fibronectin in Human Articular Cartilage," *Osteoarthritis and Cartilage* 10, no. 7 (2002): 556–63.

10. M. C. Hochberg et al., "Serum Levels of Insulin-Like Growth Factor in Subjects with Osteoarthritis of the Knee. Data from the Baltimore Longitudinal Study of Aging," *Arthritis and Rheumatism* 37, no. 8 (1994): 1177–80; S. Pagura et al., "Women Awaiting Knee Replacement Have Reduced Function and Growth Hormone," *Clinical Orthopaedics and Related Research* 415 (2003): 202–13.

11. R. A. Rogachefsky et al., "Treatment of Canine Osteoarthritis with Insulin-Like Growth Factor-1 (IGF-1) and Sodium Pentosan Polysulfate," *Osteoarthritis and Cartilage* 1, no. 2 (1993): 105–14.

12. S. B. Trippel, "Growth Factor Inhibition: Potential Role in the Etiopathogenesis of Osteoarthritis," *Clinical Orthopaedics and Related Research* 427, supp. (2004): S47–S52.

13. C. J. Malemud, N. Islam, and T. M. Haggi, "Pathophysiological Mechanisms in Osteoarthritis Lead to Novel Therapeutic Strategies," *Cells Tissues Organs* 174, no. 1–2 (2003): 34–48.

14. C. W. Denko and C. J. Malemud, "Metabolic Disturbances and Synovial Joint Responses in Osteoarthritis," *Frontiers in Bioscience* 4 (1999): D686–93.

15. G. Verbruggen, "Chondroprotective Drugs in Degenerative Joint Diseases," *Rheumatology* 45, no. 2 (2006): 129–38.

16. W. Hui, A. D. Rowan, and T. Cawston, "Insulin-Like Growth Factor 1 Blocks Collagen Release and Down Regulates Matrix Metalloproteinase-1, -3, -8, and -13 mRNA Expression in Bovine Nasal Cartilage Stimulated with Oncostatin M in Combination with Interleukin 1 Alpha," *Annals of the Rheumatic Diseases* 60 (2001): 254–61.

17. J. Stove et al., "Interleukin-1 Beta Induces Different Gene Expression of Stromelysin, Aggrecan and Tumor-Necrosis-Factor-Stimulated Gene 6 in Human Osteoarthritic Chondrocytes In Vitro," *Pathobiology* 68, no. 3 (2000): 144–49.

18. Forsyth et al., "Increased Matrix Metalloproteinase-13 Production."

19. Y. Zhong et al., "C-Reactive Protein Upregulates Receptor for Advanced Glycation End Products Expression in Human Endothelial Cells," *Hypertension* 48 (2006): 504–11.

20. Ibid.

21. P. Delerive, J. C. Fruchart, and B. Staels, "Peroxisome Proliferator-Activated Receptors in Inflammation Control," *Journal of Endocrinology* 169, no. 3 (2001): 453–59.

22. D. Moulin, "Rosiglitazone Induces Interleukin-1 Receptor Antagonist in Interleukin-1-Beta-Stimulated Rat Synovial Fibroblasts via a Peroxisome Proliferator-Activated Receptor Beta-1-Delta-Dependent Mechanism," *Arthritis and Rheumatism* 52, no. 3 (2005): 759–69.

23. K. F. Petersen and G. I. Shulman, "Etiology of Insulin Resistance," *American Journal of Medicine* 119, no. 5A (2006): 10S–16S.

24. L. Rui et al., "SOCS-1 and SOCS-3 Block Insulin Signaling by Ubiquitin-Mediated Degradation of IRS1 and IRS2," *Journal of Biological Chemistry* 277 (2002): 42394–98.

25. D. B. Savage, K. F. Petersen, and G. I. Shulman, "Mechanisms of Insulin Resistance in Humans and Possible Links With Inflammation," *Hypertension* 45 (2005): 828.

26. P. Dandona et al., "Metabolic Syndrome: A Comprehensive Perspective Based on Interactions between Obesity, Diabetes, and Inflammation," *Circulation* 111 (2005): 1448–54.

27. Xu, "Chronic Inflammation."

28. P. Libby, "Inflammation and Cardiovascular Disease Mechanisms," *American Journal of Clinical Nutrition* 83, supp. (2006): 456S–460S; A. Tedgui and Z. Mallat, "Cytokines in Atherosclerosis: Pathogenic and Regulatory Pathways," *Physiological Reviews* 86 (2006): 515–81.

29. P. Dieppe et al., "Prediction of the Progression of Joint Space Narrowing in Osteoarthritis of the Knee by Bone Scintigraphy," *Annals of the Rheumatic Diseases* 52 (1993): 557–63.

30. U. Valcourt et al., "Non-enzymatic Glycation of Bone Collagen Modifies Osteoclastic Activity and Differentiation," *Journal of Biological Chemistry* 282, no. 8 (2007): 5691–703.

31. M. Lamghari et al., "Leptin Effect on RANKL and OPG Expression in MC3T3-E1 Osteoblasts," *Journal of Cellular Biochemistry* 98, no. 5 (2006): 1123–29.

32. F. Elefteriou et al., "Leptin Regulation of Bone Resorption by the Sympathetic Nervous System and CART," *Nature* 437, no. 7032 (2005): 514–20.

33. H. Blain et al., "Serum Leptin Level Is a Predictor of Bone Mineral Density in Postmenopausal Women," *Journal of Clinical Endocrinology and Metabolism* 87, no. 3 (2002): 1030–35.

34. R. V. Considine et al., "Serum Immunoreactive Leptin Concentrations in Normal Weight and Obese Humans," *New England Journal of Medicine* 334, no. 5 (1996): 292–95.

35. D. T. Felson et al., "Bone Marrow Edema and Its Relation to Progression of Knee Osteoarthritis," *Annals of Internal Medicine* 139 (2003): 330–36.

36. T. Hayami et al., "The Role of Subchondral Bone Remodeling in Osteoarthritis: Reduction of Cartilage Degeneration and Prevention of Osteophyte Formation by Alendronate in the Rat Anterior Cruciate Ligament Transection Model," *Arthritis and Rheumatism* 50, no. 4 (2004): 1193–206; J. S. Kuliwaba et al., "Enhanced Expression of Osteocalcin mRNA in Human Osteoarthritic Trabecular Bone of the Proximal Femur Is Associated with Decreased Expression of Interleukin-6 and Interleukin-11 mRNA," *Journal of Bone and Mineral Research* 15, no. 2 (2000): 332–41.

37. A. J. Bailey et al., "Biochemical and Mechanical Properties of Subchondral Bone in Osteoarthritis," *Biorheology* 41, no. 3–4 (2004): 349–58.

38. T. J. Martin, "Paracrine Regulation of Osteoclast Formation and

Activity: Milestones in Discovery," *Journal of Musculoskeletal and Neuronal Interactions* 4, no. 3 (2004): 243–53.

39. J.-P. Pelletier et al., "The Protective Effect of Licofelone on Experimental Osteoarthritis Is Correlated with the Downregulation of Gene Expression and Protein Synthesis of Several Major Catabolic Factors: MMP-13, Cathepsin K and Aggrecanases," *Arthritis Research and Therapy* 7, no. 5 (2005): R1091–R1102.

40. D. Giugliano, A. Ceriello, and K. Esposito, "The Effects of Diet on Inflammation: Emphasis on the Metabolic Syndrome," *Journal of the American College of Cardiology* 48 (2006): 677–85.

41. L. Rui et al., "SOCS-1 and SOCS-3 Block Insulin Signaling by Ubiquitin-Mediated Degradation of IRS1 and IRS2," *Journal of Biological Chemistry* 277 (2002): 42394–98.

42. A. Aljada et al., "Glucose Intake Induces an Increase in AP-1 and Egr-1 Binding Activities and Tissue Factor and Matrix Metalloproteinase Expressions in Mononuclear Cells and Plasma Tissue Factor and Matrix Metalloproteinase Concentrations," *American Journal of Clinical Nutrition* 80 (2004): 51–57.

43. Kornman, "Interleukin 1 Genetics."

44. W.-H. Shao et al., "Targeted Disruption of Leukotriene B4 Receptors BLT1 and BLT2: A Critical Role for BLT1 in Collagen-Induced Arthritis in Mice," *Journal of Immunology* 176 (2006): 6254–61.

45. M. Hasson, "NSAIDs and COX-2 Inhibitors Impede Tendon, Bone, and Cartilage Repair," *Orthopedics Today* (September 2006) 49–50.

46. T. Ushiyama et al., "Cytokine Production in the Infrapatellar Fat Pad: Another Source of Cytokines in Knee Synovial Fluids," *Annals of the Rheumatic Diseases* 62 (2003): 108–12.

47. F. Brighenti et al., "Total Antioxidant Capacity of the Diet Is Inversely and Independently Related to Plasma Concentration of High-Sensitivity C-Reactive Protein in Adult Italian Subjects," *British Journal of Nutrition* 93, no. 5 (2005): 619–25; K. Esposito and D. Giugliano, "Diet and Inflammation: A Link to Metabolic and Cardiovascular Diseases," *European Heart Journal* 27, no 1 (2006): 15–20; Giugliano, Ceriello, and Esposito, "The Effects of Diet on Inflammation."

48. C. Chrysohoou et al., "Adherence to the Mediterranean Diet Attenuates Inflammation and Coagulation Process in Healthy Adults: The Attica Study," *Journal of the American College of Cardiology* 44 (2004): 152–58.

49. Ibid.

50. A. Trichopoulou et al., "Adherence to a Mediterranean Diet and Survival in a Greek Population," *New England Journal of Medicine* 348, no. 26 (2003): 2599–608.

51. D. Giugliano and K. Esposito, "Mediterranean Diet and Cardiovascular Health," *Annals of the New York Academy of Sciences* 1056 (2005): 253–60.

52. M. deLorgeril et al., "Mediterranean Diet, Traditional Risk Factors, and the Rate of Cardiovascular Complications after Myocardial Infarction," *Circulation* 99 (1999): 779–85.

53. K. Esposito et al., "Effect of a Mediterranean Style Diet on Endothelial Dysfunction and Markers of Vascular Inflammation in the Metabolic Syndrome: A Randomized Trial," *Journal of the American Medical Association* 292, no. 12 (2004): 1440–46.

54. K. Esposito et al., "Effect of Weight Loss and Lifestyle Changes on Vascular Inflammatory Markers in Obese Women: A Randomized Trial," *Journal of the American Medical Association* 289, no. 14 (2003): 1799–804.

55. Giugliano, Ceriello, and Esposito, "The Effects of Diet on Inflammation."

CHAPTER 9: OMEGA-3S: THE GOOD FATS THAT QUENCH THE FIRE OF INFLAMMATION

1. Z. Fan et al., "Regulation of Anabolic and Catabolic Gene Expression in Normal and Osteoarthritic Adult Human Articular Chondrocytes by Osteogenic Protein-1," *Clinical and Experimental Rheumatology* 22, no. 1 (2004): 103–106.

2. J. C. Fernandes, J. Martel-Pelletier, and J.-P. Pelletier, "The Role of Cytokines in Osteoarthritis Pathophysiology," *Biorheology* 39, nos. 1–2 (2002): 237–46.

3. C. L. Curtis et al., "Pathologic Indicators of Degradation and Inflammation in Human Osteoarthritic Cartilage Are Abrogated by Exposure to n-3 Fatty Acids," *Arthritis and Rheumatism* 46, no. 6 (2002): 1544–53; C. L. Curtis et al., "n-3 Fatty Acids Specifically Modulate Catabolic Factors Involved in Articular Cartilage Degradation," *Journal of Biological Chemistry* 275, no. 2 (2000): 721–24.

4. C. L. Curtis et al., "Effects of n-3 Fatty Acids on Cartilage Metabolism," *Proceedings of the Nutrition Society* 61, no. 3 (2002): 381–89.

5. K. D. Hankenson et al., "Omega-3 Fatty Acids Enhance Ligament Fibroblast Collagen Formation in Association with Changes in Interleukin-6 Production," *Proceedings of the Society for Experimental Biology and Medicine* 223 (2000): 88–95.

6. B. A. Watkins, L. Yong, and M. F. Seifert, "Nutraceutical Fatty Acids as Biochemical and Molecular Modulators of Skeletal Biology," *Journal of the American College of Nutrition* 20, no. 90005 (2001): 410S–416S.

7. K. Sakaguchi, I. Morita, and S. Murota, "Eicosapentanoic Acid Inhibits Bone Loss Due to Ovariectomy in Rats," *Prostaglandins Leukotrienes and Essential Fatty Acids* 50 (1994): 81–84.

8. E. Lopez-Garcia, M. B. Schulze, and J. E. Manson, "Consumption of (n-3) Fatty Acids Is Related to Plasma Biomarkers of Inflammation and Endothelial Activation in Women," *Journal of Nutrition* 134 (2004): 1806–11.

9. K. Niu et al., "Dietary Long-Chain n-3 Fatty Acids of Marine Origin and Serum C-Reactive Protein Concentrations Are Associated in a Population with a Diet Rich in Marine Products," *American Journal of Clinical Nutrition* 84, no. 1 (2006): 223–29; T. Pischon et al., "Habitual Dietary Intake of n-3 and n-6 Fatty Acids in Relation to Inflammatory Markers among U.S. Men and Women," *Circulation* 108 (2003): 155; L. Ferrucci et al., "Relationship of Plasma Polyunsaturated Fatty Acids to Circulating Inflammatory Markers," *Journal of Clinical Endocrinology and Metabolism* 91, no. 2 (2006): 439–46; F. B. Hu et al., "Fish and Long Chain Omega-3 Fatty Acid Intake and Risk of Coronary Heart Disease and Total Mortality in Diabetic Women," *Circulation* 107 (2003): 1852–57; F. B. Hu and W. C. Willett, "Optimal Diets for Prevention of Coronary Heart Disease," *Journal of the American Medical Association* 288 (2002): 2569–78; B. M. Rasmussen et al., "Effects of Dietary Saturated, Monounsaturated, and n-3 Fatty Acids on Blood Pressure in Healthy Subjects," *American Journal of Clinical Nutrition* 83 (2006): 221–26.

10. C. Klein-Platat et al., "Plasma Fatty Acid Composition Is Associated with the Metabolic Syndrome and Low-Grade Inflammation in Overweight Adolescents," *American Journal of Clinical Nutrition* 82 (2005): 1178–84.

CHAPTER 10: UNHEALTHY DIETS CAUSE HORMONAL IMBALANCE

1. A. Schaffler et al., "Role of Adipose Tissue as an Inflammatory Organ in Human Diseases," *Endocrine Reviews* 27, no. 5 (2006): 449–67; M. Otero, R. Lago, and R. Gomez, "Towards a Pro-inflammatory and Immunomodulatory Emerging Role of Leptin," *Rheumatology* 45 (2006): 944–50; A. Schaffler et al., "Adipocytokines in Synovial Fluid," *Journal of the American Medical Association* 290, no. 13 (2003): 1709–10.

2. Otero, Lago, and Gomez, "Towards a Pro-inflammatory and Immunomodulatory Emerging Role of Leptin"; F. M. H. Van Dielen et al., "Leptin and Soluble Leptin Receptor Levels in Obese and Weight-Losing Individuals," *Journal of Clinical Endocrinology and Metabolism* 87, no. 4 (2002): 1708–16.

3. G. Matarese et al., "Leptin as a Novel Therapeutic Target for Immune Intervention," *Current Drug Targets—Inflammation and Allergy* 1, no. 1 (2002): 13–22.

4. J.-N. Huan et al., "Adipocyte-Selective Reduction of the Leptin Receptors Induced by Antisense RNA Leads to Increased Adiposity, Dyslipidemia, and Insulin Resistance," *Journal of Biological Chemistry* 278, no. 46 (2003): 45638–50.

5. H. Bays, L. Mandarino, and R. A. DeFronzo, "Role of the Adipocyte, Free Fatty Acids, and Ectopic Fat in Pathogenesis of Type 2 Diabetes Mellitus: Peroxisomal Proliferator-Activator Receptor Agonists Provide a Rational Therapeutic Approach," *Journal of Clinical Endocrinology and Metabolism* 89, no. 2 (2004): 463–78.

6. R. V. Considine et al., "Serum Immunoreactive Leptin Concentrations in Normal Weight and Obese Humans," *New England Journal of Medicine* 334, no. 5 (1996): 292–95.

7. J. F. Caro et al., "Decreased Cerebrospinal Fluid/Serum Leptin Ratio in Obesity: A Possible Mechanism for Leptin Resistance," *Lancet* 348, no. 9021 (1996): 159–61.

8. C. A. Meier et al., "IL-1 Receptor Antagonist Serum Levels Are Increased in Human Obesity: A Possible Link to the Resistance of Leptin?" *Journal of Clinical Endocrinology and Metabolism* 87, no. 3 (2002): 1184–88; G. Boden et al., "Effects of Prolonged Hyperinsulinemia on Serum

Leptin in Normal Human Subjects," *Journal of Clinical Investigation* 100, no. 5 (1997): 1107–13.

9. C. M. Morberg et al., "Leptin and Bone Mineral Density: A Cross-Sectional Study in Obese and Nonobese Men," *Journal of Clinical Endocrinology and Metabolism* 88, no. 12 (2003): 5795–800.

10. M. Otero et al., "Leptin, from Fat to Inflammation: Old Questions and New Insights," *FEBS Letter* 579, no. 2 (2005): 295–301.

11. M. Otero, J. J. Gomez-Reino, and O. Gualillo, "Synergistic Induction of Nitric Oxide Synthase Type II: In Vitro Effect of Leptin and Interferon-Gamma in Human Chondrocytes and ATDC5 Chondrogenic Cells," *Arthritis and Rheumatism* 48, no. 2 (2003): 404–409.

12. J. P. Koshy et al., "The Modulation of Matrix Metalloproteinase and ADAM Gene Expression in Human Chondrocytes by Interleukin-1 and Oncostatin M: A Time-Course Study Using Real-Time Quantitative Reverse Transcription-Polymerase Chain Reaction," *Arthritis and Rheumatism* 46 (2002): 961–67.

13. Y. Figenschau et al., "Human Articular Chondrocytes Express Functional Leptin Receptors," *Biochemical and Biophysical Research Communications* 287, no. 1 (2001): 190.

14. M. Morroni et al., "In Vivo Leptin Expression in Cartilage and Bone Cells of Growing Rats and Adult Humans," *Journal of Anatomy* 205, no. 4 (2004): 291.

15. H. Dumond et al., "Evidence of a Key Role of Leptin in Osteoarthritis," *Arthritis and Rheumatism* 48, no. 11 (2003): 3118–29.

16. Ibid.

17. Ibid.

18. A. J. Teichtahl et al., "Obesity and Female Sex, Risk Factors for Knee Osteoarthritis That May Be Attributable to Systemic or Local Leptin Biosynthesis and Its Cellular Effects," *Medical Hypotheses* 65, no. 2 (2005): 312–15; R. Weiss et al., "Low Adiponectin Levels in Adolescent Obesity: A Marker of Increased Intramyocellular Lipid Accumulation," *Journal of Clinical Endocrinology and Metabolism* 88, no. 5 (2003): 2014–18.

19. T. Kadowaki et al., "Adiponectin and Adiponectin Receptors in Insulin Resistance, Diabetes, and the Metabolic Syndrome," *Journal of Clinical Investigation* 116 (2006): 1784–92.

20. Y. Yamamoto et al., "Adiponectin, and Adipocyte-Derived Protein, Predicts Future Insulin Resistance: Two-Year Followup Study in Japanese

Population," *Journal of Clinical Endocrinology and Metabolism* 89, no. 1 (2004): 87–90; A. Ehling et al., "The Potential of Adiponectin in Driving Arthritis," *Journal of Immunology* 176 (2006): 4468–78.

21. U. Muller-Ladner et al., "The Potential Role of Adiponectin in Driving Arthritis," *Arthritis Research and Therapy* 6, supp. 3 (2004): 63.

22. M. G. Jeschke et al., "Insulin Attenuates the Systemic Inflammatory Response in Endotoxemic Rats," *Endocrinology* 145 (2004): 4084–93.

23. P. Dandona, "Inflammation: The Link between Insulin Resistance, Obesity and Diabetes," *Trends in Immunology* 25 (2004): 4–7.

24. X. Chen et al., "Association of Glutathione Peroxidase Activity with Insulin Resistance and Dietary Fat Intake during Normal Pregnancy," *Journal of Clinical Endocrinology and Metabolism* 88, no. 12 (2003): 5963–68.

25. P. Gillery, "Oxidative Stress and Protein Glycation in Diabetes Mellitus," *Annales de Biologie Clinique* 64, no. 4 (2006): 309–14; J. Yangsoo et al., "Association of the 276(G-T) Polymorphism of the Adiponectin Gene with Cardiovascular Disease Risk Factors in Nondiabetic Koreans," *American Journal of Clinical Nutrition* 82 (2005): 760–67.

26. Teichtahl et al., "Obesity and Female Sex."

27. Ibid.

28. D. T. Felson et al., "Weight Loss Reduces the Risk for Symptomatic Knee Osteoarthritis in Women: The Framingham Study," *Annals of Internal Medicine* 116, no. 7 (1992): 535–39.

29. Ibid.

30. B. Boyan, "Estrogen Receptors in Cartilage." Arthritis Research Conference, Keystone, Colorado, June 26–29, 2003.

31. C. Ding et al., "Knee Structural Alteration and BMI: A Cross-Sectional Study," *Obesity Research* 13 (2005): 350–61; Y. Zhang et al., "Bone Mineral Density and Risk of Incident and Progressive Radiographic Knee Osteoarthritis in Women: The Framingham Study," *Journal of Rheumatology* 27, no. 4 (2000): 1032–37.

32. T. M. D'Eon et al., "Estrogen Regulation of Adiposity and Fuel Partitioning: Evidence of Genomic and Non-genomic Regulation of Lipogenic and Oxidative Pathways," *Journal of Biological Chemistry* 280, no. 43 (2005): 35983–91.

CHAPTER 11: SWEET TOXINS THAT DESTROY OUR JOINTS: HOW AGEs LEAD TO OSTEOARTHRITIS

1. L. J. Sandell and T. Aigner, "Articular Cartilage and Changes in Arthritis. An Introduction: Cell Biology of Osteoarthritis," *Arthritis Research* 3, no. 2 (2001): 107–13.

2. D. L. Cecil et al., "Inflammation-Induced Chondrocyte Hypertrophy Is Driven by Receptor for Advanced Glycation End Products," *Journal of Immunology* 175, no. 12 (2005): 8296–302.

3. M. M. C. Steenvoorden, PhD thesis, Department of Rheumatology, Faculty of Medicine/Leiden University Medical Center (LUMC), Leiden University, Netherlands, 2007; J. DeGroot et al., "Age-Related Disease in Proteoglycan Synthesis in Human Articular Chondrocytes: The Role of Nonenzymatic Glycation," *Arthritis and Rheumatism* 42, no. 5 (1999): 1003–1009.

4. J. R. Chen et al., "Comparison of the Concentrations of Pentosidine in the Synovial Fluid, Serum and Urine of Patients with Rheumatoid Arthritis and Osteoarthritis," *Rheumatology* 38 (1999): 1275–78; L. Senolt et al., "Increased Pentosidine, an Advanced Glycation End Product, in Serm and Synovial Fluid from Patients with Knee Osteoarthritis and Its Relation with Cartilage Oligomeric Matrix Protein," *Annals of the Rheumatic Diseases* 64 (2005): 886–90.

5. R. Ramasamy et al., "Advanced Glycation End Products and RAGE: A Common Thread in Aging, Diabetes, Neurodegeneration, and Inflammation," *Glycobiology* 15, no. 7 (2005): 16R–28R.

6. Z. Alikhani et al., "Advanced Glycation End Products Enhance Expression of Pro-apoptotic Genes and Stimulate Fibroblast Apoptosis through Cytoplasmic and Mitochondrial Pathways," *Journal of Biological Chemistry* 280, no. 13 (2005): 12087–95.

7. J. DeGroot et al., "Accumulation of Advanced Glycation End Products as a Molecular Mechanism for Aging as a Risk Factor for Osteoarthritis," *Arthritis and Rheumatism* 50, no. 4 (2004): 1207–15; M. Takahashi, "Pentosidine, an Advanced Glycation End Product, and Arthritis," *Current Rheumatology Reviews* 2, no. 4 (2006): 319–24; N. Verzijl et al., "Crosslinking by Advanced Glycation End Products Increases

the Stiffness of the Collagen Network in Human Articular Cartilage: A Possible Mechanism through Which Age Is a Risk Factor for Osteoarthritis," *Arthritis and Rheumatism* 46 (2002): 114–23; H. K. Pokharna et al., "Lysyl Oxidase and Maillard Reaction-Mediated Cross Links in Aging and Osteoarthritic Rabbit Cartilage," *Journal of Orthopaedic Research* 13, no. 1 (1995): 13–21.

8. DeGroot et al., "Accumulation of Advanced Glycation End Products."

9. T. Chavakis, A. Bierhaus, and P. P. Nawroth, "RAGE (Receptor for Advanced Glycation End Products): A Central Player in the Inflammatory Response," *Microbes and Infection* 6, no. 13 (2004): 1219–25.

10. M.-P. Wautier et al., "Activation of NADPH Oxidase by AGE Links Oxidant Stress to Altered Gene Expression via RAGE," *American Journal of Physiology, Endocrinology and Metabolism* 280 (2001): E685–E694.

11. G. Ferreti et al., "Glycated Low-Density Lipoproteins Modify Platelet Properties: A Compositional and Functional Study," *Journal of Clinical Endocrinology and Metabolism* 87, no. 5 (2002): 2180–84.

12. C. Weijng et al., "High Levels of Dietary Advanced Glycation End Products Transform Low-Density Lipoprotein into a Potent Redox-Sensitive Mitogen-Activated Protein Kinase Stimulant in Diabetic Patients," *Circulation* 110 (2004): 285–91.

13. T. Goldberg et al., "Advanced Glycoxidation End Products in Commonly Consumed Foods," *Journal of the American Dietetic Association* 104, no. 8 (2004): 1287–91.

14. H. Vlassara and M. R. Palace, "Diabetes and Advanced Glycation End Products," *Journal of Internal Medicine* 251, no. 2 (2002): 87–101.

15. DeGroot et al., "Accumulation of Advanced Glycation End Products."

16. M. M. Steenvoorden et al., "Activation of Receptor for Advanced Glycation End Products in Osteoarthritis Leads to Increased Stimulation of Chondrocytes and Synoviocytes," *Arthritis and Rheumatism* 54, no. 1 (2006): 14–18.

17. R. F. Loeser et al., "Articular Chondrocytes Express the Receptor for Advanced Glycation End Products: Potential Role in Osteoarthritis," *Arthritis and Rheumatism* 52, no. 8 (2005): 2376–85.

18. Chavakis, Bierhaus, and Nawroth, "RAGE (Receptor for Advanced Glycation End Products)."

19. H. M. Lander et al., "Activation of the Receptor for Advanced Gly-

cation End Products Triggers a p21ras-Dependent Mitogen-Activated Protein Kinase Pathway Regulated by Oxidant Stress," *Journal of Biological Chemistry* 272, no. 28 (1997): 17810–14.

20. R. K. M. Wong et al., "Advanced Glycation End Products Stimulate an Enhanced Neutrophil Respiratory Burst Mediated through the Activation of Cytosolic Phospholipase A2 and Generation of Arachidonic Acid," *Circulation* 108 (2003): 1858.

21. Ibid.

22. M. A. Hofmann et al., "RAGE and Arthritis: The G82S Polymorphism Amplifies the Inflammatory Response," *Genes and Immunity* 3, no. 3 (2002): 123–35.

23. Ibid.

24. Z. Zhou et al., "Regulation of Osteoclast Function and Bone Mass by RAGE," *Journal of Experimental Medicine* (2005): 1067–80; T. Miyata et al., "Advanced Glycation End Products Enhance Osteoclast-Induced Bone Resorption in Cultured Mouse Unfractionated Bone Cells and in Rats Implanted Subcutaneously with Devitalized Bone Particles," *Journal of the American Society of Nephrology* 8 (1997): 260–70.

CHAPTER 12: WHY IT IS NOT A GOOD IDEA TO TREAT OSTEOARTHRITIS WITH DRUGS

1. B. J. deVries et al., "Effects of NSAIDs on the Metabolism of Sulphated Glycosaminoglycans in Healthy and (Post) Arthritic Murine Articular Cartilage," *Drugs* 35, no. 1 (1988): 24–32; J. T. Dingle, "The Effects of NSAID on the Matrix of Human Articular Cartilages," *Zeitschrift fur Rheumatologie* 58, no. 3 (1999): 125–29.

2. M. R. Griffin et al., "Non-steroidal Anti-inflammatory Drug Use and Increased Risk of Peptic Ulcer Disease in Elderly Persons," *Annals of Internal Medicine* 114, no. 4 (1991): 257–63.

3. C. Knouff and J. Auwerx, "Peroxisome Proliferator-Activated Receptor-Gamma Calls for Activation in Moderation: Lessons from Genetics and Pharmacology," *Endocrine Reviews* 25, no. 6 (2004): 899–918.

4. S. A. Maher et al., "What's New in Orthopedic Research," *Journal of Bone and Joint Surgery* 88-A, no. 10 (2006): 2314–21.

5. D. Stickens et al., "Altered Endochondral Bone Development in Matrix Metalloproteinase 13-Deficient Mice," *Development* 131 (2004): 5883–95.

6. J.-O. Deguchi et al., "Matrix Metalloproteinase-13/Collagenase-3 Deletion Promotes Collagen Accumulation and Organization in Mouse Atherosclerotic Plaques," *Circulation* 112 (2005): 2708–15.

7. K. D. Brandt et al., "OA-Doxycycline Study Group. Doxycycline (Doxy) Slows the Rate of Joint Space Narrowing (JSN) in Patients with Knee Osteoarthritis (OA)," Presented at the American College of Rheumatology Annual Meeting, Orlando Florida, 2003, abstract #SLB22.

8. G. M. Mutlu et al., "Pulmonary Adverse Events of Anti-Tumor Necrosis Factor-alpha Antibody Therapy," *American Journal of Medicine* 119 (2006): 639–46.

9. T. Bongartz et al., "Anti-TNF antibody Therapy in Rheumatoid Arthritis and the Risk of Serious Infections and Malignancies: Systematic Review and Meta-Analysis of Rare Harmful Effects in Randomized Controlled Trials," *Journal of the American Medical Association* 295 (2006): 2275–85.

10. Ibid.

11. J. Askling et al., "Hematopoietic Malignancies in Rheumatoid Arthritis: Lymphoma Risk and Characteristics after Exposure to Tumor Necrosis Factor Antagonists," *Annals of the Rheumatic Diseases* 64 (2005): 1414–20.

12. H. Komuro et al., "The Osteoprotegerin/Receptor Activator of Nuclear Factor Kappa B/Receptor Activator of Nuclear Factor Kappa B Ligan System in Cartilage," *Arthritis and Rheumatism* 44, no. 12 (2001): 2768–76.

13. N. Presle et al., "Cartilage Protection by Nitric Oxide Synthase Inhibitors after Intra-Articular Injection of Interleukin-1Beta in Rats," *Arthritis and Rheumatism* 42, no. 10 (1999): 2094–102.

14. Maher et al., "What's New in Orthopedic Research."

15. D. Geroldi, C. Falcone, and E. Enzo, "Soluble Receptor for Advanced Glycation End Products: From Disease Marker to Potential Therapeutic Target," *Current Medicinal Chemistry* 13, no. 17 (2006): 1971–78.

16. V. P. Reddy and A. Beyaz, "Inhibitors of the Maillard Reaction and AGE Breakers as Therapeutics for Multiple Diseases," *Drug Discovery Today* 11, no. 13–14 (2006): 646–54.

17. S.-B. Woo, K. Hande, and P. G. Richardson, "Osteonecrosis of the Jaw and Biphosphonates," *New England Journal of Medicine* 353 (2005): 100.

CHAPTER 13: NEW GENETIC RESEARCH IS UNRAVELING THE MYSTERIES OF OSTEOARTHRITIS

1. K. S. Kornman, "Interleukin 1 Genetics, Inflammatory Mechanisms and Nutrigenic Opportunities to Modulate Diseases of Aging," *American Journal of Clinical Nutrition* 83, supp. (2006): 475S–483S.

2. C. A. Cooney, A. A. Dave, and G. L. Wolff, "Maternal Methyl Supplements in Mice Affect Epigenetic Variation and DNA Methylation of Offspring," *Journal of Nutrition* 132 (2002): 2393S–2400S.

3. M. Fenech, "Micronutrients and Genomic Stability: A New Paradigm for Recommended Daily Allowances (RDAs)," *Food and Chemical Toxicology* 40, no. 8 (2002): 1113–17.

4. B. N. Ames, "DNA Damage from Micronutrient Deficiencies Is Likely to Be a Major Cause of Cancer," *Mutation Research* 475 (2001): 7–20; B. N. Ames, "Micronutrient Deficiencies: A Major Cause of DNA Damage," *Annals of the New York Academy of Sciences* 889 (1999): 87–106.

5. Fenech, "Micronutrients and Genomic Stability"; Cooney, Dave, and Wolff, "Maternal Methyl Supplements in Mice."

6. C. B. Forsyth et al., "Increased Matrix Metalloproteinase-13 Production with Aging by Human Articular Chondrocytes in Response to Catabolic Stimuli," *Journals of Gerontology Series A: Biological Sciences and Medical Sciences* 60, no. 9 (2005): 1118–24.

7. J.-P. Pelletier et al., "The Protective Effect of Licofelone on Experimental Osteoarthritis Is Correlated with the Downregulation of Gene Expression and Protein Synthesis of Several Major Catabolic Factors: MMP-13, Cathepsin K and Aggrecanases," *Arthritis Research and Therapy* 7, no. 5 (2005): R1091–R1102.

8. Ibid.

9. H. Stanton et al., "ADAMTS 5 Is the Major Aggrecanase in Mouse Cartilage In Vivo and In Vitro," *Nature* 434, no. 7033 (2005): 648–52.

10. M. D. Kofron and C. T. Laurencin, "Orthopaedic Applications of Gene Therapy," *Current Gene Therapy* 5, no. 1 (2005): 37–61.

11. P. E. DiCesare et al., "Regional Gene Therapy for Full-Thickness Articular Cartilage Lesions Using Naked DNA with a Collagen Matrix," *Journal of Orthopedic Research* 24, no. 5 (2006): 1118–27.

12. G. W. Duff, "Evidence for Genetic Variation as a Factor in Maintaining Health," *American Journal of Clinical Nutrition* 83, supp. (2006): 431S–435S; C. H. Evans et al., "Osteoarthritis Gene Therapy," *Gene Therapy* 11, no. 4 (2004): 379–89.

13. L. S. Lohmander and D. Felson, "Can We Identify a 'High Risk' Patient Profile to Determine Who Will Experience Rapid Progression of Osteoarthritis?" *Osteoarthritis and Cartilage* 12, supp. A (2004): 549–52; V. B. Kraus, "Biomarkers in Osteoarthritis," *Current Opinion in Rheumatology* 17, no. 5 (2005): 641–46; S. Christgau and P. A. C. Cloos, "Cartilage Degradation Products as Markers for Evaluation of Patients with Rheumatic Disease," *Clinical and Applied Immunology Reviews* 4, no. 4 (2004): 277–94.

14. C. Klein-Platat et al., "Plasma Fatty Acid Composition Is Associated with the Metabolic Syndrome and Low-Grade Inflammation in Overweight Adolescents," *American Journal of Clinical Nutrition* 82 (2005): 1178–84.

15. M. Ricote et al., "The Peroxisome Proliferator-Activated Receptor-Gamma Is a Negative Regulator of Macrophage Activation," *Nature* 391, no. 6662 (1998): 79–82.

16. R. K. Berge et al., "The Metabolic Syndrome and the Hepatic Fatty Acid Drainage Hypothesis," *Biochimie* 87, no. 1 (2005): 15–20; P. Ferre, "The Biology of Peroxisome Proliferator-Activated Receptors: Relationship with Lipid Metabolism and Insulin Sensitivity," *Diabetes* 53 (2004): S43–S50.

17. C. Knouff and J. Auwerx, "Peroxisome Proliferator-Activated Receptor-Gamma Calls for Activation in Moderation: Lessons from Genetics and Pharmacology," *Endocrine Reviews* 25, no. 6 (2004): 899–918.

18. J. I. Pulai et al., "NFkappaB Mediates the Stimulation of Cyokine and Chemokine Expression by Human Articular Chondrocytes in Response to Fibronectin Fragments," *Journal of Immunology* 174 (2005): 5781–88.

CHAPTER 14: BENEFICIAL NUTRIENTS FOR JOINTS

1. M. A. Flynn, W. Irwin, and G. Krause. "The Effect of Folate and Cobalamin on Osteoarthritic Hands," *Journal of the American College of Nutrition* 13, no. 4 (1994): 351–56.

2. B. N. Ames, L. S. Gold, and W. C. Willett, "The Causes and Prevention of Cancer," *Proceedings of the National Academy of Sciences of the United States of America* 92 (1995): 5258–65; B. N. Ames and L. S. Gold, "Endogenous Mutagens and the Causes of Aging and Cancer," *Mutation Research* 250 (1991): 3–16; B. N. Ames, "Micronutrients Prevent Cancer and Delay Aging," *Toxicology Letter* 102–103 (1998): 5–18.

3. M. J. Gibney and R. Gibney, "Diet, Genes and Disease: Implications for Nutrition Policy," *Proceedings of the Nutrition Society* 63 (2003): 491–500.

4. Homocysteine Lowering Trialist's Collaboration, "Dose-Dependent Effects of Folic Acid on Blood Concentrations of Homocysteine: A Meta-analysis of the Randomized Trials," *American Journal of Clinical Nutrition* 82 (2005): 806–12.

5. W. B. Jonas, C. P. Rapoza, and W. F. Blair, "The Effect of Niacinamide on Osteoarthritis: A Pilot Study," *Inflammation Research* 45, no. 7 (1996): 330–34.

CHAPTER 15: THE NUTRACEUTICAL ARSENAL NEEDED TO COMBAT OSTEOARTHRITIS

1. L. M. Stead et al., "Is It Time to Re-evaluate Methyl Balance in Humans?" *American Journal of Clinical Nutrition* 83 (2006): 5–10.

2. D. J. Stott et al., "Randomized Controlled Trial of Homocysteine-Lowering Vitamin Treatment in Elderly Patients with Vascular Disease," *American Journal of Clinical Nutrition* 82 (2005): 1320–26.

3. W. I. Najm et al., "S-Adenosyl Methionine (SAMe) versus Celecoxib for the Treatment of Osteoarthritis Symptoms," *BMC Musculoskeletal Disorders* 5 (2004): 6.

4. C. DiPadova, "S-Adenosylmethionine in the Treatment of

Osteoarthritis. Review of the Clinical Studies," *American Journal of the Medical Sciences* 83, no. 5A (1987): 60–65.

5. H. A. Barcelo et al., "Effect of S-Adenosyl Methionine on Experimental Osteoarthritis in Rabbits," *American Journal of the Medical Sciences* 83, no. 5A (1987): 55–59.

6. B. Konig, "A Long-Term (Two Years) Clinical Trial with S-Adenosyl Methionine for the Treatment of Osteoarthritis," *American Journal of the Medical Sciences* 83, no. 5A (1987): 89–94.

7. G. Vetter, "Double-Blind Comparative Clinical Trial with S-Adenosyl Methionine and Indomethacin in the Treatment of Osteoarthritis," *American Journal of the Medical Sciences* 83, no. 5A (1987): 78–80.

8. A. Maccagno et al., "Double-Blind Controlled Clinical Trial of Oral S-Adenosyl Methionine versus Piroxicam in Knee Osteoarthritis," *American Journal of the Medical Sciences* 83, no. 5A (1987): 72–77.

9. H. Muller-Fassenbender, "Double-Blind Clinical Trial of S-Adenosyl Methionine versus Ibuprofen in the Treatment of Osteoarthritis," *American Journal of the Medical Sciences* 83, no. 5A (1987): 81–83.

10. Homocysteine Lowering Trialist's Collaboration, "Dose-Dependent Effects of Folic Acid on Blood Concentrations of Homocysteine: A Meta-analysis of the Randomized Trials," *American Journal of Clinical Nutrition* 82 (2005): 806–12.

11. V. Ganji and M. R. Kafai, "Frequent Consumption of Milk, Yogurt, Cold Breakfast Cereals, Peppers, and Cruciferous Vegetables and Intakes of Dietary Folate and Riboflavin but Not Vitamins B-12 and B-6 Are Inversely Associated with Serum Total Homocysteine Concentrations in the U.S. Population," *American Journal of Clinical Nutrition* 80 (2004): 1500–507.

12. R. E. Newnham, "Essentiality of Boron for Healthy Bones and Joints," *Environmental Health Perspectives* 102, supp. 7 (1994): 83–85.

13. Ibid.

14. S. Sasaki et al., "Low-Selenium Diet, Bone, and Articular Cartilage in Rats," *Nutrition* 10, no. 6 (1994): 538–43.

15. Y. E. Henroitin et al., "Avocado/Soybean Unsaponifiables Increase Aggrecan Synthesis and Reduce Catabolic and Pro-inflammatory Mediator Production by Human Osteoarthritic Chondrocytes," *Journal of Rheumatology* 30 (2003): 1825–34.

16. E. Maheu et al., "Symptomatic Efficacy of Avocado/Soybean Unsaponifiables in the Treatment of Osteoarthritis of the Knee and Hip: A

Prospective, Randomized, Double-Blind, Placebo-Controlled, Multicenter Clinical Trial with a Six Month Treatment Period and a Two-Month Follow-up Demonstrating a Persistent Effect," *Arthritis and Rheumatism* 41, no. 1 (1998): 81–91.

17. M. A. Cake et al., "Modification of Articular Cartilage and Subchondral Bone Pathology in an Ovine Meniscectomy Model of Osteoarthritis by Avocado and Soya Unsaponifiables (ASU)," *Osteoarthritis and Cartilage* 8, no. 6 (2000): 404–11.

18. B. H. Arjmandi et al., "Soy Protein May Alleviate Osteoarthritis Symptoms," *Phytomedicine* 11 (2004): 567–75.

19. J. A. Martin et al., "Chondrocyte Senescence, Joint Loading and Osteoarthritis," *Clinical Orthopedics and Related Research* 427, supp. (2004): S96–S103.

20. N. Elmali et al., "Effect of Resveratrol in Experimental Osteoarthritis in Rabbits," *Inflammation Research* 54, no. 4 (2005): 158–62.

21. R. Estruch et al., "Different Effects of Red Wine and Gin Consumption on Inflammatory Biomarkers of Atherosclerosis: A Prospective Randomized Crossover Trial. Effect of Wine on Inflammatory Markers," *Atherosclerosis* 175 (2004): 117–23.

22. M. Demeule et al., "Matrix Metalloproteinase Inhibition by Green Tea Catechins," *Biochimica Et Biophysica Acta* 1478, no. 1 (2000): 51–60.

23. S. Elliott et al., "The Triterpenoid CDDO Inhibits Expression of Matrix Metalloproteinase-1, Matrix Metalloproteinase-13 and Bcl-3 in Primary Human Chondrocytes," *Arthritis Research and Therapy* 5, no. 5 (2003): R285–R291.

24. S. M. Henning et al., "Bioavailability and Antioxidant Activity of Tea Flavanols after Consumption of Green Tea, Black Tea, or a Green Tea Extract Supplement," *American Journal of Clinical Nutrition* 80 (2004): 1558–64.

25. S. Ahmed, "Green Tea Polyphenol Epigallocatechin-3-Gallate Inhibits the IL-1-Beta-Induced Activity and Expression of Cyclooxygenase-2 and Nitric Oxide Synthase-2 in Human Chondrocytes," *Free Radical Biology and Medicine* 33, no. 8 (2002): 1097–102.

26. J. L. Evans et al., "Oxidative Stress and Stress-Activated Signaling Pathways: A Unifying Hypothesis of Type 2 Diabetes," *Endocrine Reviews* 23, no. 5 (2002): 599–622.

27. P. Peristeris et al., "N-Acetylcysteine and Glutathione as Inhibitors of Tumor Necrosis Factor Production," *Cellular Immunology* 140, no. 2 (1992):

390–99; G. Wu, Y.-Z. Fang, and S. Yang, "Glutathione Metabolism and Its Implications for Health," *Journal of Nutrition* 134 (2004): 489–92.

28. O. I. Aruoma et al., "The Antioxidant Action of N-Acetylcysteine: Its Reaction with Hydrogen Peroxide, Hydroxyl Radical, Superoxide, and Hypochlorous Acid," *Free Radical Biology and Medicine* 6, no. 6 (1989): 593–97; M. Zafarullah et al., "Molecular Mechanisms of N-Acetylcysteine Actions," *Cellular and Molecular Life Sciences* 6, no. 1 (2003): 6–20; S. Bergamini et al., "N-Acetylcysteine Inhibitors in Vivo Nitric Oxide Production by Inducible Nitric Oxide Synthase," *Nitric Oxide: Biology and Chemistry* 5, no. 4 (2001): 349–60.

29. M. Thomson et al., "Including Garlic in the Diet May Help Lower Blood Glucose, Cholesterol, and Triglycerides," *Journal of Nutrition* 136, no. 3 (2006): 800S–802S.

30. J. Pleiner et al., "FFA-Induced Endothelial Dysfunction Can Be Corrected by Vitamin C," *Journal of Clinical Endocrinology and Metabolism* 87, no. 6 (2002): 2913–17.

31. A. E. Fletcher, E. Breeze, and P. Shetty, "Antioxidant Vitamins and Mortality in Older Persons—Findings from the Nutrition Add-On Study to the Medical Research Council Trial of Assessment and Management of Older People in the Community," *American Journal of Clinical Nutrition* 78 (2003): 999–1010.

32. T. E. McAlindon et al., "Do Antioxidant Micronutrients Protect against the Development and Progression of Knee Osteoarthritis," *Arthritis and Rheumatism* 39, no. 4 (1996): 648–56.

33. A. G. Clark et al., "The Effects of Ascorbic Acid on Cartilage Metabolism in Guinea Pig Articular Cartilage Explants," *Matrix Biology* 21, no. 2 (2002): 175–84.

34. N. H. Jensen, "Reduced Pain from Osteoarthritis in Hip Joint or Knee Joint during Treatment with Calcium Ascorbate. A Randomized, Placebo-Controlled Cross-Over Trial in General Practice," *Ugeskrift For Laeger* 165 (2003): 2563–66.

35. J. A. Martin et al., "Effects of Oxidative Damage and Telomerase Activity on Human Articular Cartilage Chondrocyte Senescence," *Journals of Gerontology Series: A Biological Sciences and Medical Sciences* 59 (2004): B324–B336.

36. G. Kaiki et al., "Osteoarthritis Induced by Intra-articular Hydrogen

Peroxide Injection and Running Load," *Journal of Orthopedic Research* 8, no. 5 (1990): 731–40.

37. Ibid.

38. G. Blankenhorn, "Clinical Effectiveness of Spondyvit (Vitamin E) in Activated Arthroses," *Zeitschrift Fur Orthopadie Und Ihre Grenzgebiete* 124, no. 3 (1986): 340–43.

39. O. Scherak et al., "High-Dosage Vitamin E Therapy in Patients with Activated Arthrosis," *Zeitschrift Fur Rheumatologie* 49, no. 6 (1990): 369–73.

40. T. E. McAlindon et al., "Relation of Dietary Intake and Serum Levels of Vitamin D to Progression of Osteoarthritis of the Knee among Participants in the Framingham Study," *Annals of Internal Medicine* 125, no. 5 (1996): 353–59.

41. Ibid.

42. N. E. Lane et al., "Serum Vitamin D Levels and Incident Changes of Radiographic Hip Osteoarthritis: A Longitudinal Study," *Arthritis and Rheumatism* 42, no. 5 (1999): 854–60.

43. T. Stammers, B. Sibbald, and P. Freeling, "Fish Oil in Osteoarthritis," *Lancet* 2, no. 8661 (1989): 503.

44. C. L. Curtis et al., "n-3 Fatty Acids Specifically Modulate Catabolic Factors Involved in Articular Cartilage Degradation," *Journal of Biological Chemistry* 275, no. 2 (2000): 721–24.

45. S. Jacob et al., "Oral Administration of RAC-Alpha-Lipoic Acid Modulates Insulin Sensitivity in Patients with Type 2 Diabetes Mellitus: A Placebo Controlled Pilot Trial," *Free Radical Biology and Medicine* 27 (1999): 309–14.

46. T. M. Hagen et al., "Mitochondrial Decay in the Aging Rat Heart: Evidence for Improvement by Dietary Supplementation with Acetyl-L-Carnitine and/or Lipoic Acid," *Annals of the New York Academy of Sciences* 959 (2002): 491–507.

47. J. Liu et al., "Memory Loss in Old Rats Is Associated with Brain Mitochondrial Decay and RNA/DNA Oxidation: Partial Reversal by Feeding Acetyl-L-Carnitine and/or R-Alpha-Lipoic Acid," *Proceedings of the National Academy of Sciences of the United States of America* 99, no. 4 (2002): 2356–61.

48. T. M. Hagen et al., "Feeding Acetyl-L-Carnitine and Lipoic Acid to Old Rats Significantly Improves Metabolic Function While Decreasing

Oxidative Stress," *Proceedings of the National Academy of Sciences of the United States of America* 99, no. 4 (2002): 1870–75.

49. T. M. Hagen et al., "®-Alpha-Lipoic Acid-Supplemented Old Rats Have Improved Mitochondrial Function, Decreased Oxidative Damage, and Increased Metabolic Rate," *FASEB Journal* 13 (1999): 411–18.

50. P. S. Chan et al., "Glucosamine and Chondroitin Sulfate Regulate Gene Expression and Synthesis of Nitric Oxide and Prostaglandin E(2) in Articular Cartilage Explants," *Osteoarthritis and Cartilage* 13, no. 5 (2005): 387–94.

51. J. Y. Reginster et al., "Long-Term Effects of Glucosamine Sulphate on Osteoarthritis Progression: A Randomized, Placebo-Controlled Clinical Trial," *Lancet* 357, no. 9252 (2001): 251–56.

52. J. P. Rindone et al., "Randomized Controlled Trial of Glucosamine for Treating Osteoarthritis of the Knee," *Western Journal of Medicine* 172, no. 2 (2000): 91–94.

53. K. Pavelka et al., "Glucosamine Sulfate Use and Delay of Progression of Knee Osteoarthritis," *Archives of Internal Medicine* 162, no. 18 (2002): 2113–23.

54. T. E. McAlindon et al., "Effectiveness of Glucosamine for Symptoms of Knee Osteoarthritis: Results from an Internet-Based Randomized Double-Blind Controlled Trial," *American Journal of Medicine* 117, no. 9 (2004): 643–49.

55. G. X. Giu et al., "Efficacy and Safety of Glucosamine Sulfate versus Ibuprofen in Patients with Knee Osteoarthritis," *Arzneimittel Forschung/Drug Research* 48, no. 5 (1998): 469–74.

56. W. Noack et al., "Glucosamine Sulfate in Osteoarthritis of the Knee," *Osteoarthritis and Cartilage* 2, no. 1 (1994): 51–59.

57. A. Reichelt et al., "Efficacy and Safety of Intramuscular Glucosamine Sulfate in Osteoarthritis of the Knee. A Randomised, Placebo-Controlled, Double-Blind Study," *Arzneimittel Forschung/Drug Research* 44, no. 1 (1994): 75–80.

58. P. R. Usha and M. U. R. Naidu, "Randomised, Double-Blind, Parallel, Placebo-Controlled Study of Oral Glucosamine, Methylsulfonylmethane and their Combination in Osteoarthritis," *Clinical Drug Investigation* 24, no. 6 (2004): 353–63.

59. T. E. McAlindon et al., "Glucosamine and Chondroitin for Treatment

of Osteoarthritis: A Systematic Quality Assessment and Meta-Analysis," *Journal of the American Medical Association* 283, no. 11 (2000): 1469–75.

60. T. Conrozier, "Anti-arthrosis Treatments: Efficacy and Tolerance of Chondroitin Sulfates (CS 4+6)," *Presse Medicale* 27, no. 36 (1998): 1862–65.

61. B. Mazieres et al., "Chondroitin Sulfate in the Treatment of Gonarthrosis and Coxarthrosis. 5-Months Result of a Multicenter Double-Blind Controlled Prospective Study Using Placebo," *Revue du Rhumatisme et des Maladies Osteo-Articulaires* 59, no. 7–8 (1992): 466–72.

62. P. Morreale et al., "Comparison of the Anti-inflammatory Efficacy of Chondroitin Sulfate and Diclofenac Sodium in Patients with Knee Osteoarthritis," *Journal of Rheumatology* 23, no. 8 (1996): 1385–91.

63. B. A. Michel et al., "Chondroitins 4 and 6 Sulfate in Osteoarthritis of the Knee: A Randomized, Controlled Trial," *Arthritis and Rheumatism* 52, no. 3 (2005): 779–86.

64. P. Mathieu, "A New Mechanism of Action of Chondroitin Sulfates ACS4-ACS6 in Osteoarthritic Cartilage," *Presse Medicale* 31, no. 29 (2002): 1383–85.

65. B. F. Leeb et al., "A Meta-analysis of Chondroitin Sulfate in the Treatment of Osteoarthritis," *Journal of Rheumatology* 27, no. 1 (2000): 205–11.

CHAPTER 16: DIETARY RECOMMENDATIONS IN OSTEOARTHRITIS FOR THE NEW MILLENNIUM

1. F. Brighenti et al., "Total Antioxidant Capacity of the Diet Is Inversely and Independently Related to Plasma Concentration of High-Sensitivity C-Reactive Protein," *British Journal of Nutrition* 93, no. 5 (2005): 619–25; B. Watzl et al., "A 4-Week Intervention with High Intake of Carotenoid-Rich Vegetables and Fruit Reduces Plasma C-Reactive Protein in Healthy, Non-smoking Men," *American Journal of Clinical Nutrition* 82 (2005): 1052–58.

2. K. Esposito et al., "Effect of a Mediterranean-Style Diet on Endothelial Dysfunction and Markers of Vascular Inflammation in the Metabolic

Syndrome: A Randomized Trial," *Journal of the American Medical Association* 292 (2004): 1440–46.

3. A. Basu, S. Devaraj, and I. Jialal, "Dietary Factors That Promote or Retard Inflammation," *Arteriosclerosis, Thrombosis, and Vascular Biology* 26 (2006): 995.

4. H. Bliddal and R. Christensen, "The Management of Osteoarthritis in the Obese Patient: Practical Considerations and Guidelines for Therapy," *Obesity Reviews Online Early*, July 18, 2006.

5. S. P. Messier et al., "Exercise and Dietary Weight Loss in Overweight and Obese Older Adults with Knee Osteoarthritis: The Arthritis, Diet, and Activity Promotion Trial," *Arthritis and Rheumatism* 50, no. 5 (2004): 1501–10.

CHAPTER 17: WHY WE NEED A PARADIGM SHIFT IN MEDICINE

1. T. Kuhn, *The Structure of Scientific Revolutions*, 2nd ed. (Chicago: University of Chicago Press, 1970).

2. Ibid.

3. A. Donabedian, *The Definition of Quality and Approaches to Its Assessment* (Ann Arbor, MI: Health Administration Press, 1980).

4. J. Carey, "Medical Guesswork: From Heart Surgery to Prostate Care, the Health Industry Knows Little about Which Common Treatments Really Work," *Business Week*, May 2006, 73–79.

CHAPTER 18: LOOKING TO THE FUTURE

1. M. Gebauer et al., "Repression of Anti-proliferative Factor Tob1 in Osteoarthritic Cartilage," *Arthritis Research and Therapy* 7 (2005): R274–R284.

2. P. J. Stover, "Influence of Human Genetic Variation on Nutritional Requirements," *American Journal of Clinical Nutrition* 83, supp. (2006): 436S–442S.

3. J. M. Ordovas, "Genetic Interactions with Diet Influence the Risk of

Cardiovascular Disease," *American Journal of Clinical Nutrition* 83, supp. (2006): 443S–446S.

4. K. S. Kornman, "Interleukin 1 Genetics, Inflammatory Mechanisms and Nutrigenetic Opportunities to Modulate Diseases of Aging," *American Journal of Clinical Nutrition* 83, supp. (2006): 475S–483S.

5. Ibid.

6. Y. Gafni et al., "Stem Cells as Vehicles for Orthopedic Gene Therapy," *Gene Therapy* 11, no. 4 (2004): 417–26.

7. M. J. Gibney, "Nutrigenomics in Human Nutrition—An Overview," *South African Journal of Clinical Nutrition* 18, no. 2 (2005): 115–18.

8. J. Luan et al., "Evidence for Gene-Nutrient Interaction at the PPAR Gamma Locus," *Diabetes* 50 (2001): 686–89.

9. R. Gobezie et al., "Proteomics: Applications to the Study of Rheumatoid Arthritis and Osteoarthritis," *Journal of the American Academy of Orthopedic Surgeons* 14, no. 6 (2006): 325–32.

10. P. E. DiCesare et al., "Localization and Expression of Cartilage Oligomeric Matrix Protein by Human Rheumatoid and Osteoarthritic Synovium and Cartilage," *Journal of Orthopedic Research* 17, no. 3 (1999): 437–45.

11. Gibney, "Nutrigenomics in Human Nutrition."

12. J. B. German, M.-A. Roberts, and S. M. Watkins, "Personal Metabolomics as a Next-Generation Nutritional Assessment," *Journal of Nutrition* 133 (2003): 4260–66.

13. R.-J. Lamers et al., "Identification of Disease-and Nutrient-Related Metabolic Fingerprints in Osteoarthritic Guinea Pigs," *Journal of Nutrition* 133 (2003): 1776–80.

14. S. M. Watkins and J. B. German, "Toward the Implementation of Metabolomic Assessments of Human Health and Nutrition," *Current Opinion in Biotechnology* 13 (2002): 512–16.

Index

277